Dorsaf Makhlouf
Nahla Kechiche Sahnoun
Lassaad Sahnoun

Lung sequestration in children

Dorsaf Makhlouf
Nahla Kechiche Sahnoun
Lassaad Sahnoun

Lung sequestration in children

Bronchopulmonary malformation

ScienciaScripts

Imprint

Cover image: www.ingimage.com

This book is a translation from the original published under ISBN 978-620-6-72218-2.

Publisher:
Sciencia Scripts
is a trademark of
Dodo Books Indian Ocean Ltd. and OmniScriptum S.R.L publishing group

120 High Road, East Finchley, London, N2 9ED, United Kingdom
Str. Armeneasca 28/1, office 1, Chisinau MD-2012, Republic of Moldova, Europe
Printed at: see last page
ISBN: 978-620-8-19860-2

Contents

1 INTRODUCTION....2
2 MATERIALS AND METHODS....3
3 RESULTS....35
APPENDIX....69
References....71

1 INTRODUCTION

Pulmonary sequestration (PS) is a bronchopulmonary malformation corresponding to a segment of the lung that does not communicate with the tracheobronchial tree and has systemic arterial vascularisation [1,2]. The term sequestration was introduced by Pryce in 1946 and is derived from the Latin sequestrae, meaning "to separate" [3,4].

It is a rare condition, accounting for 0.15-6.5% of lung malformations [2,5,6].

There are two types of pulmonary sequestration [7,8]:

- SIL: 75%.
- SEL: 25% DISCOUNT

Despite the development of antenatal and postnatal diagnostic techniques, MS continues to pose a number of problems:

- The etiopathogeny remains obscure.
- The clinical and radiological signs are variable and non-specific, and may be responsible for diagnostic and therapeutic errors.
- Therapeutic management, both antenatal and postnatal, remains controversial.
- The existence of a number of hybrid forms is a surprise which further complicates the etiopathogeny, clinical course and treatment.

This demonstrates the value of our study in describing the clinical and radiological factors that enable the diagnosis of pulmonary sequestration.

The objectives of this work are to :

- clarify the embryological, etiopathological and anatomopathological aspects of pulmonary sequestration,
- study the epidemiological and clinical features,
- explain the elements of radiological diagnosis,
- comparing the diagnoses suggested on imaging with the results of the pathological examination,
- discuss the different approaches to lung sequestration surgery in children,
- and discuss the diagnostic problems that may arise with other congenital or acquired conditions.

2 MATERIALS AND METHODS

This work is based on a retrospective descriptive study of 16 observations of pulmonary sequestration treated in the paediatric surgery department of the Fattouma Bourguiba Hospital in Monastir. These observations were collected over a period of 29 years, from January 1990 to December 2019.

The positive diagnosis was confirmed by the anatomopathological findings.

A data collection form was drawn up and included epidemiological, clinical, paraclinical, therapeutic and developmental data.

- appendix 1). Information was collected from hospital records and operative and pathology reports.

Patients were called in to discuss their long-term course and have a chest X-ray.

Observation 1:

Infant (T.F), aged 1 and a half years; male, born at term by Caesarean section from a non-consanguineous manage. The mother had had 7 pregnancies: 3 parites and 4 abortions. The pregnancy progressed normally. Obstetric ultrasound at 16 weeks' gestation revealed cystic pulmonary images suggestive of cystic adenomatoid malformation of the left lung, with no impact on lung or fetal growth.

At birth, the physical examination was normal; Apgar: 9/10, PN: 3kg400, no respiratory symptoms were noted.

On admission, the interview revealed no pathological antecedents and no medication taken during pregnancy.

The physical examination was normal, with no abnormalities on pulmonary examination.

A chest X-ray showed a left basi-thoracic pulmonary condensation with compensatory hypertrophy of the right lung.

Thoracic computed tomography (figure 1) showed an irregular left lower lobar mass with a dual tissue component of homogeneous enhancement, and a cystic mass formed by three macrocysts varying in size from 12 to 16mm. The mass measured 36 x 24 mm axially and extended to 32 mm in height. There was also a left posterobasal parenchymal condensation containing an aerial bronchogram and vascularised by a systemic artery originating in the left lateral wall of the descending thoracic aorta and measuring 5mm in diameter.

The diagnosis was cystic adenomatoid malformation corresponding to the left lower lobar mass associated with posterobasal intra-lobar pulmonary sequestration.

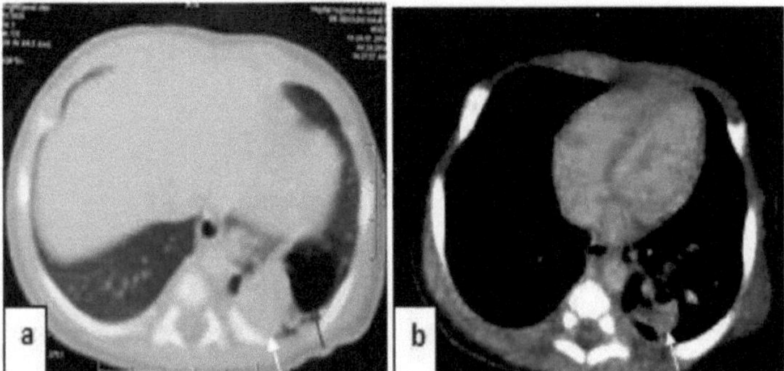

Fig.1(a,b): Axial section thoracic CT in parenchymal window (a) mediastinal (b) showing the left posterobasal cystic mass (red arrow) and the parenchymal condensation at its contact (white arrow) vascularised by an artery originating from the thoracic aorta (green arrow).

The infant was operated on thoracoscopically. A first 5 mm trocar was inserted below the scapula, at the intersection between the anterior axillary line and the 5[eme] intercostal space. A pneumathorax was created by insufflation of CO2 (pressure of 8 millimetres of mercury). Two other 5mm operating trocars were placed in triangulation and behind the axillary line. Intraoperative exploration revealed multiple adhesions between the left lower lobe and the chest wall. Dissection of these adhesions revealed an artery arising from the descending aorta and vascularising the pulmonary sequestration. An attempt to electrosect this artery failed, with uncontrollable bleeding, and the decision was made to convert to thoracotomy. Vascular ligation was performed. A left inferior lobectomy was performed, including sequestration and placement of a chest drain. The post-operative course was straightforward. The chest tube was removed at 3 days post-operatively. The patient was discharged after five days. Histological examination showed cystic pockets lined with pseudostratified ciliated columnar epithelium. The systemic vessel was of the arterial type. This was consistent with intra-lobar pulmonary sequestration associated with adenomatoid cystic malformation of the lung.

The post-operative course was straightforward, with no respiratory symptoms. The follow-up was 4 years.

Observation 2:

A male infant (B.C), aged 45 days, diagnosed antenatally with a large left pleural effusion, was born at term by cesarean section to a primiparous mother. The patient was admitted immediately postnatally for respiratory distress related to his left pleural effusion, requiring mechanical ventilation for 10 days.

The chest X-ray showed water opacity covering the whole of the left pulmonary hemichamber, with compression of the mediastinum (Figure 2).

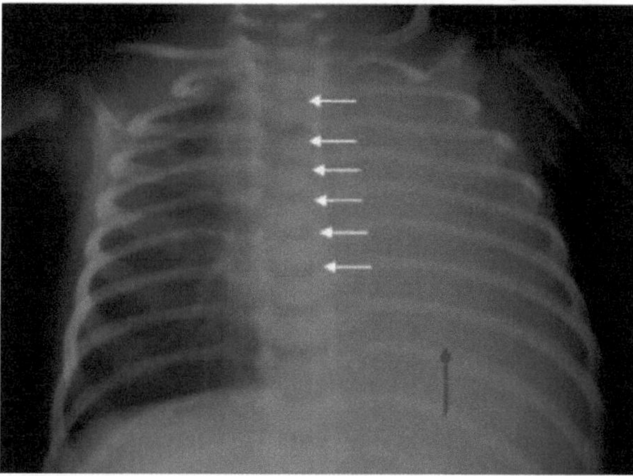

Fig.2: Front chest X-ray: Large left pleural effusion (red arrow) with mediastinum backflow towards the contralateral side (white arrows).

An initial pleural puncture yielded serohematic fluid, with the lung returning to the wall, as seen on chest X-ray. However, the revolution was marked by recurrence and worsening of the left pleural effusion, leading to a state of permanent respiratory distress.

A second pleural puncture yielded a gelatinous fluid.

A bronchopulmonary malformation was suspected, despite the fact that the thoracic ultrasound and CT scan did not reveal a cystic image with the presence of an enclosed pleura, which meant that thoracoscopic exploration was indicated.

Intraoperative examination revealed a large left pleural effusion with a lemon-yellow appearance and some loose adhesions. There was also a left basal parenchymal mass independent of the lung. It was decided to convert to thoracotomy. The lung tissue was extra-lobar and was vascularised by a large systemic vessel originating from the left lung.

abdominal stage (Figure 3). We opted for ligation of the feeding artery with exeresis of the pulmonary sequestration. Finally, the pleural cavity was drained using a N°12 tube, which was removed at 5 days post-operatively.

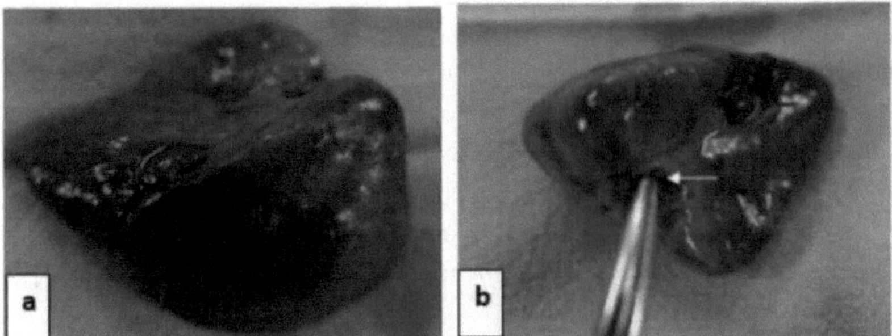

Fig.3: Sequestrectomy operative specimen showing the systemic vessel held by the forceps (arrow)

The post-operative course was straightforward. Histological examination confirmed the diagnosis, showing lung tissue rich in bronchiolar structures and arterial-type vessels. This appearance was compatible with the diagnosis of extra-lobar sequestration. The child was doing well with good respiratory status. The follow-up was 17 years.

Observation 3:

Female infant (B.K), 1 month old, born at term to a primiparous mother. Morphological ultrasound was performed at 21 days' gestation and showed a hyperechogenic mediastinal mass, located anterior to and in contact with the ascending aorta and posterior to the creur, initially suggestive of a middle

mediastinal teratoma.
At birth, the physical examination was normal. A chest X-ray revealed posterior mediastinal opacity in the retro-cardiac region (Figure 4).

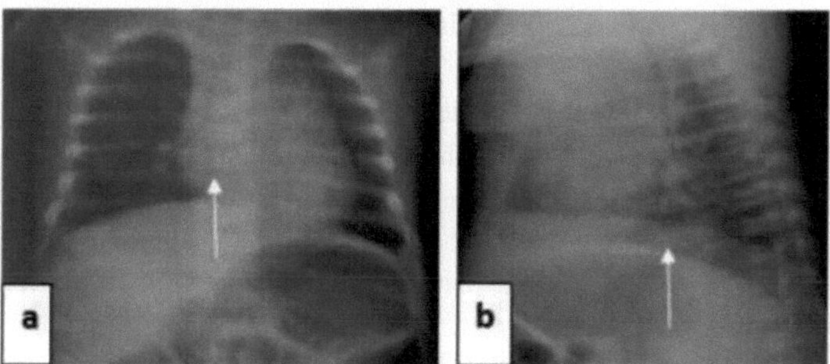

Fig.4(a,b): Front (a) and side (b) chest X-ray showing posterior mediastinal opacity (white arrows).

A thoracic angioscan performed at 20 days of age showed a right-lateral mid mediastinal tissue formation with clear contours measuring 24*19*14mm. The mass was markedly enhanced, discreetly heterogeneous with no calcifications and no fatty or necrotic component. It was fed by a systemic artery originating in the creiliac trunk and extending into the thorax through the right triangular ligament of the lung. Venous drainage was via a vein that emptied into the spleno-mesaraic trunk. This scanned appearance was mainly suggestive of right extra-lobar pulmonary sequestration.
The infant was operated on thoracoscopically. Exploration revealed a pinkish formation covered by a clean mediastinal pleura with its own vascularisation suggestive of extra-lobar pulmonary sequestration. The vascular pedicle was electrocoagulated and ligated. The surgical specimen was extracted through the trocar port. Anatomopathological examination confirmed the diagnosis of extra-lobar sequestration. The post-operative course was straightforward. The chest tube was removed at 4 days post-operatively. The patient is doing well with no respiratory signs. The follow-up is 7 years.
Comment N°4:
Female infant (K.S), 45 days old, with a history of prematurity of 33 weeks' amenorrhoea and a neonatal weight of 2650 grams, having been hospitalised at birth for neonatal respiratory distress requiring mechanical ventilation.
A fetal MRI performed at 30 days' gestation showed a right inferior lobar malformation associated with a homolateral pleural effusion suggestive of intra-lobar sequestration or cystic adenomatoid malformation. Subsequent morphological ultrasound showed a worsening of the homolateral pleural effusion with the appearance of a small peritoneal effusion.

A thoracic ultrasound performed on Day 1 of life showed a large free right pleural effusion with multiple basal right pulmonary cystic lesions associated with hypertrophy of the entire right lung. After puncture of the effusion, it recurred (Figure 5), necessitating placement of a left pleural drain, which remained in place for 6 days. Cardiac ultrasound was without abnormalities. A thoracic angioscan was ordered, and showed a large right pleural effusion, with the mediastinum backing up towards the contralateral side (Figure 6). There was also an intra-thoracic right mass, located between the right lower lobe and the homolateral diaphragmatic dome, measuring 34 x 43 x 30mm. This mass was vascularised by a systemic artery arising from the terminal portion of the descending thoracic aorta.

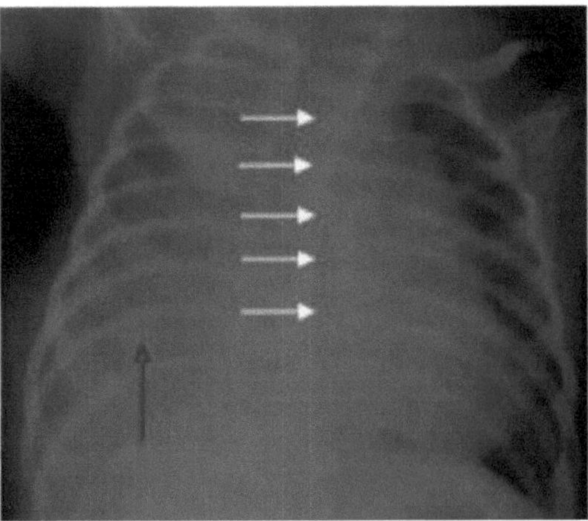

Fig.5: Front chest X-ray: large right pleural effusion (red arrow) with mediastinum backflow towards the contralateral side (white arrows).

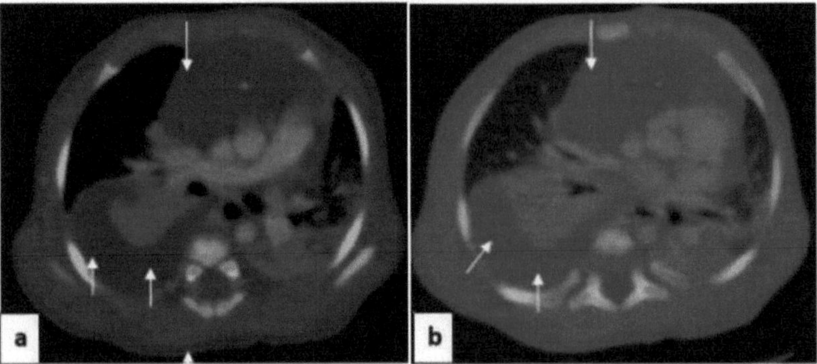

Fig.6(a,b): Axial section thoracic CT scan in mediastinal (a) and parenchymal (b) windows showing a large right pleural effusion (white arrows) with deviation of the mediastinum to the left (red arrows).

The infant underwent a right thoracotomy in the 5eme intercostal space. Exploration revealed multiple pleural adhesions, particularly in the right lower lobe. There was also a right basi-thoracic parenchymal formation, independent of the lung, covered by its own pleura and vascularised by an artery arising from the thoracic aorta. This was a right extra-lobar sequestration (Figure 7). We therefore opted for sequestrectomy with placement of a chest drain.

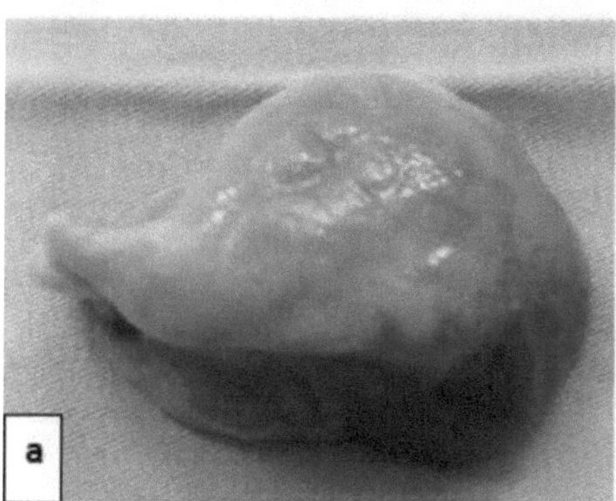

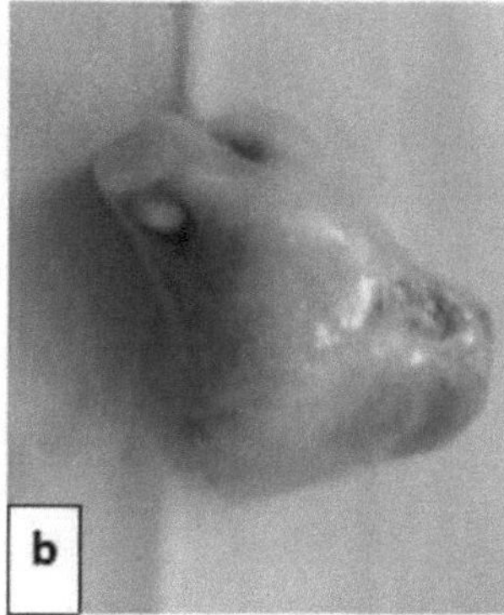

Fig.7 : Sequestrectomy operative part

On sectioning, the surgical specimen was spongy in appearance, measuring 4.5 cm in diameter.

On histology, the vessels identified on the specimen were of the arterial type. The lung parenchyma showed dilatation of the bronchioles and alveolar lumina, which in places contained macrophages.

This lesion was consistent with right extra-lobar pulmonary sequestration.

The post-operative course was straightforward. The chest tube was removed at 3 days post-operatively. The patient is doing well with no respiratory problems. The follow-up is 2 years.

Observation 5:

NRS (B.M), female, 6 months old, from a normal pregnancy, with a history of an episode of bronchoalveolitis treated as an outpatient with good progression, presented a week before her consultation with a cough and dyspnoea evolving in a febrile context.

On pulmonary auscultation, the vesicular murmurs were diminished on the right. Biological tests showed a hyperleukocytosis of 11,700/mm^3 and a CRP of 34 mg/ml.

The chest X-ray showed a large, hollow opacity with a hydro-aerobic level occupying the entire right lung field.

A thoracic CT scan showed a voluminous fluid collection in the right hemi thorax measuring 100x60x80mm, with a clean wall that was raised after injection of contrast. This collection had a drainage bronchus (right lower lobar bronchus). It exerted a significant mass effect, pushing back the mediastinum and right lung parenchyma. In addition, there was a 2eme fluid cystic formation, homogeneous, unilocular, in the posterior mediastinum, with a thin wall measuring 30 mm long (Figure 8,9).

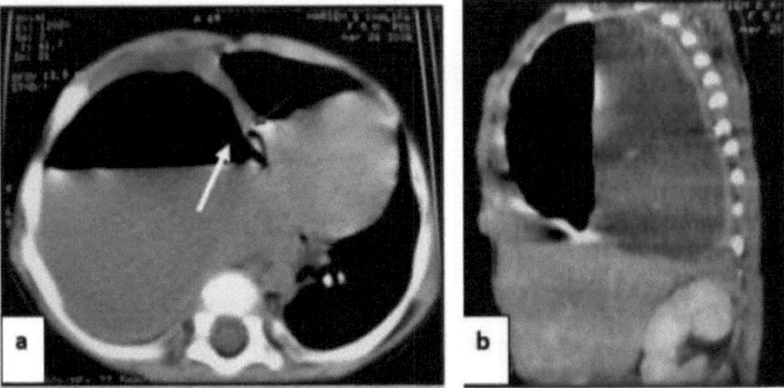

Fig.8(a,b): Chest CT scan showing a hydro-aenic collection in the right niemi-thorax (white arrows) with drainage bronchus (red arrow).

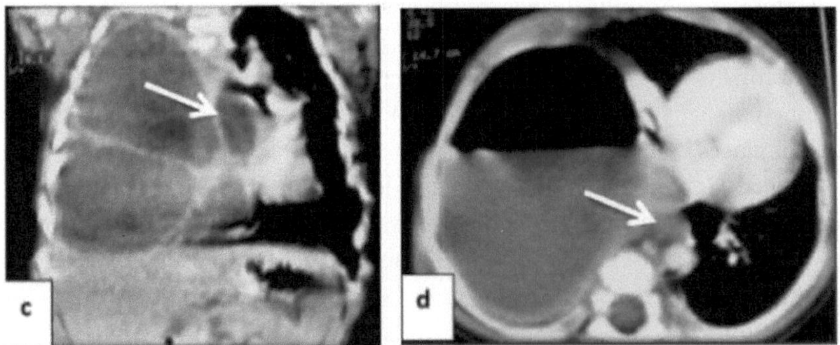

Fig.9(a,b): CT scan of the thorax showing a posterior mediastinal cystic mass (white arrows).

The infant was started on intravenous antibiotics. A radiographic check was carried out 15 days later, showing complete emptying of the hydro-aerosic collection, which had been replaced by a voluminous clara occupying the whole of the right lung field (Figure 10).

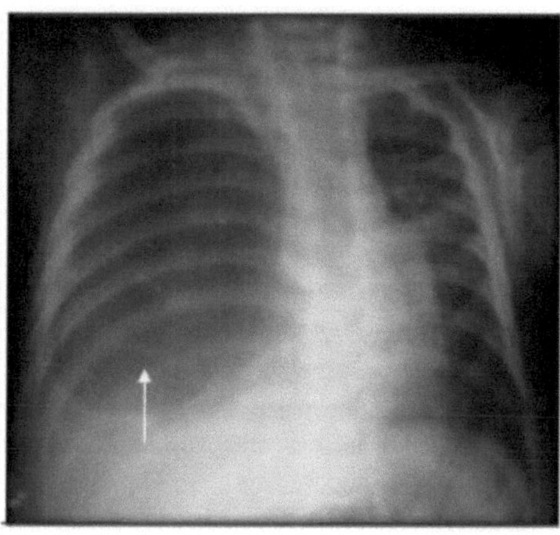

Fig.10: Front thoracic X-ray showing a voluminous clart^ of the right h6mi- lung field (white arrow)

A bronchopulmonary malformation was suspected and surgical treatment was planned.

Intraoperative examination revealed a right lower lobe with a cystic formation, the macroscopic appearance of which ë initially suggested a macrocystic pulmonary cystic adenomatoid malformation. Elsewhere, exploration revealed a right basal parenchymal mass independent of the lung suggestive of right extra-lobar pulmonary sequestration fed by a systemic artery, and another cystic formation in the posterior mediastinum not communicating with the esophagus ë suggestive of a bronchogenic cyst (figure n°11). The infant had a right inferior lobectomy, resection of the pulmonary sequestration and mediastinal bronchogenic cyst.

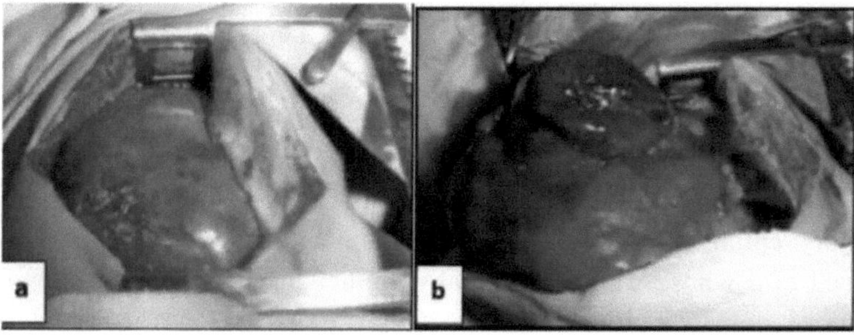

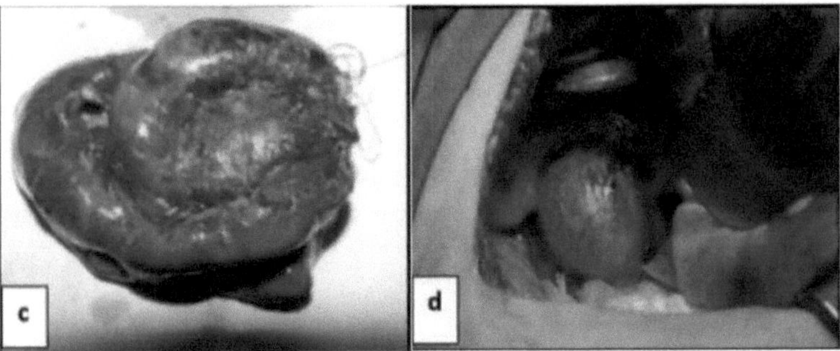

Fig.11(a,b,c,d): (a,b): Intraoperative appearance / c: Lobectomy specimen for right lower lobar MAKP / d: mediastinal bronchogenic cyst and extra-lobar sequestration

The post-operative course was straightforward, with removal of the chest tube on D11 post-op, and the infant was handed over to his parents the following day. The chest X-ray on discharge showed good lung expansion (Figure 12).

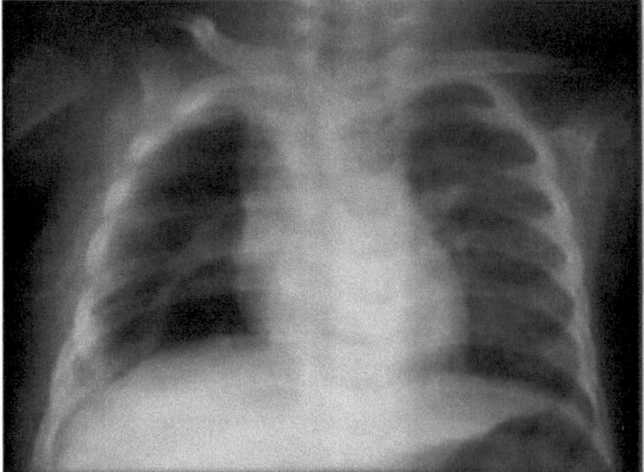

Fig.12:Post-operative radiological check: good lung expansion

Histologically, several samples were taken and showed that the wall of the cystic parenchymal formation was made up of fibrous tissue bordered by granulation tissue rich in neo-vessels and a polymorphous inflammatory infiltrate. On a single sample, the cystic wall appeared to be lined with respiratory epithelium. This cystic formation could correspond either to an abscessed cyst whose wall was partially epithelialised, probably following its communication with a bronchiole, or to a type I MAKP.

The mediastinal cyst corresponded to a bronchogenic cyst. Its wall was lined with epithelium of the respiratory type.

The third sample corresponded to extra-lobar pulmonary sequestration.

It was in the shape of a lung lobule measuring 40 x30x10mm, greyish in colour on section and with a vascular lumen 4mm in diameter. Histologically, the specimen contained numerous cysts of varying size. The interstitial tissue showed an abundant lymphocytic and plasma cell infiltrate, as well as several arterial vessels. This histopathological appearance was consistent with right pulmonary sequestration associated with a type I adenomatoid malformation and a cyst of the primary intestine.

The follow-up was 12 years. At the last clinical check-up, the patient was asymptomatic and the follow-up chest X-ray was without abnormalities.

Comment 6:

NRS (M.M), male, aged 19 months, who presented 2 months prior to hospitalisation with bronchoalveolitis, treated with antibiotics.

A chest X-ray showed left retro-cardiac opacity.

Radiological examination after 15 days of antibiotic treatment revealed the following

persistence of the same image (figure 13) .

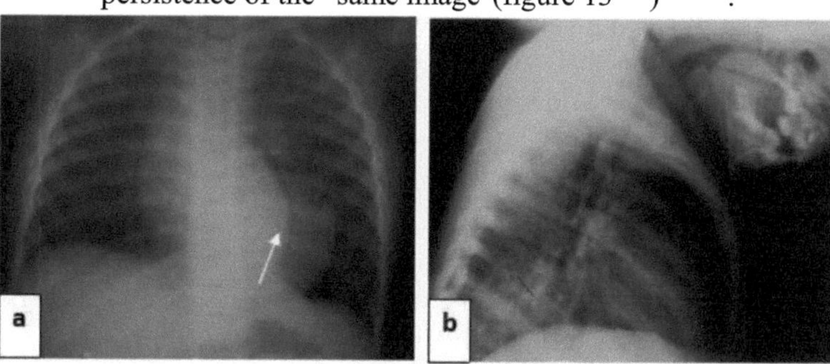

Fig.13(a,b): Chest X-ray, front (a) and side (b), showing left retrocardiac opacity (white arrow) with filling of the retrocardiac clear space (red arrow).

A thoracic CT scan (figure 14) showed a cystic formation in the left costo-vertebral gutter with close contact with the resophagus, suggestive of a bronchogenic cyst, a pleuro-pericardial cyst or a resophageal duplication.

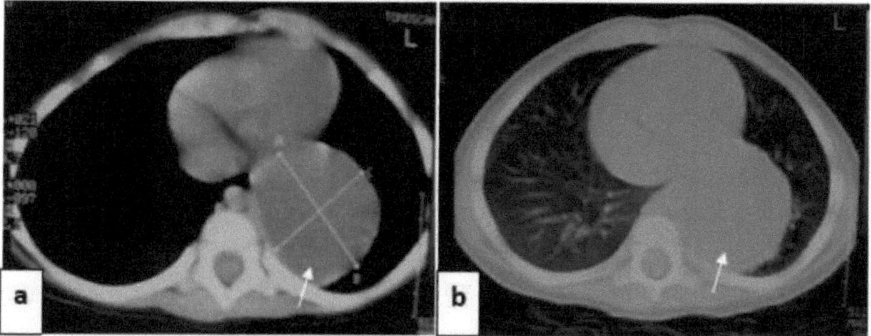

Fig.14(a,b): Chest CT in mediastinal (a) and pulmonary (b) windows showing a cystic image siëging at the level of the left доиШёге costo-vertebral (white arrows).

The child underwent thoracoscopic surgery. Exploration revealed a left mediastinal mass in close contact with the resophagus, with puncture yielding lemon-yellow fluid. Given the difficulty of thoracoscopic dissection, it was decided to convert to thoracotomy. The meticulous dissection freed a mass intimately adherent to the resophagus and the right and left pneumogastric nerves and fed by a systemic adenoma. Drainage was ensured by two thoracic drains. The post-operative course was straightforward and the infant was handed over to his parents at 5 days post-operatively after removal of the 2 drains.
Macroscopic examination revealed a thin-walled, brownish cyst 40mm in diameter. Histologically, the cyst wall was lined by epithelium which was often abraded. When preserved, it took on a cylindrical or cubic, basophilic, squamous appearance and in some places a mucinous appearance. This epithelium was supported by a dense, sparsely cellular connective tissue, which in some areas included a strip of smooth muscle tissue. In some areas, there were cavities that closely resembled bronchial tubes, as they were lined with epithelium of the respiratory type. These cavities were surrounded by bundles of smooth muscle cells with cartilaginous hotspots and bronchial-type seromucosal acinar glands. They were associated with structures reminiscent of pulmonary alveoli.
Anatomopathological examination concluded that the bronchopulmonary malformation had the appearance of an extra-lobar sequestration. This was the site of a cyst of the primitive intestine with an appearance intermediate between a bronchogenic cyst and a resophageal duplication.
The patient progressed favourably. The follow-up chest X-ray showed no abnormalities. The follow-up was 15 years.

Comment 7:

NRS (B.M), aged 9 months, male, was born at term by vaginal delivery to a primigravida primiparous mother. The pregnancy progressed normally.
Obstetric ultrasound at 16 days' gestation showed a hyperechogenic mass in the left hemi thorax. A fetal MRI (Figure 15) was performed at 23 days' gestation and showed hypersignal T2 lung parenchyma in the left hemi thorax, with identification of a vascular structure arising from the thoracic aorta and deviation of the mediastinum towards the contralateral side. In addition, the left upper lobe and right lung were normal. This appearance was suggestive of pulmonary sequestration.

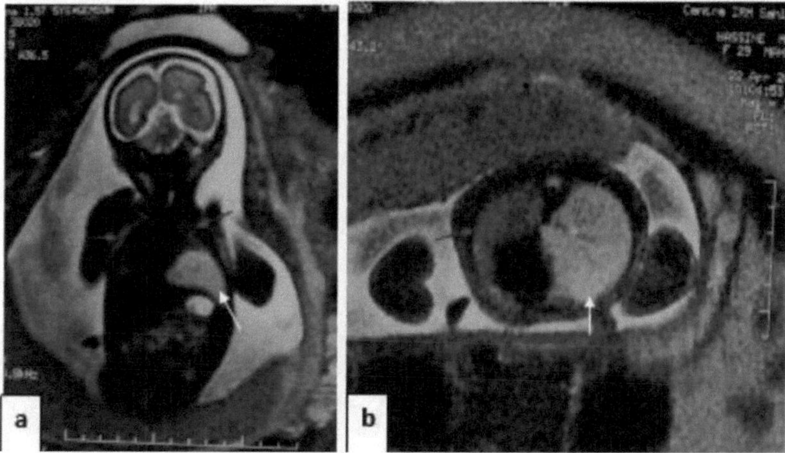

Fig.15(a,b): Fetal MRI in T2 coronal (a) and T2 axial (b) slices showing hyper signal in the left lower lobe (white arrows) with normal signal in the left upper lobe and right lung field (red arrows).

The baby was delivered at term by vaginal delivery. At birth, Apgar:9/10; PN: 3kg 500. Clinical examination revealed a systolic murmur associated with postnatal valvular pulmonary narrowing.

In addition, there was a decrease in vesicular murmurs on the left side in relation to her antenatally diagnosed bronchopulmonary malformation.

The rest of the examination was unremarkable.

The chest X-ray (Figure 16) showed a left lower parenchymal condensation.

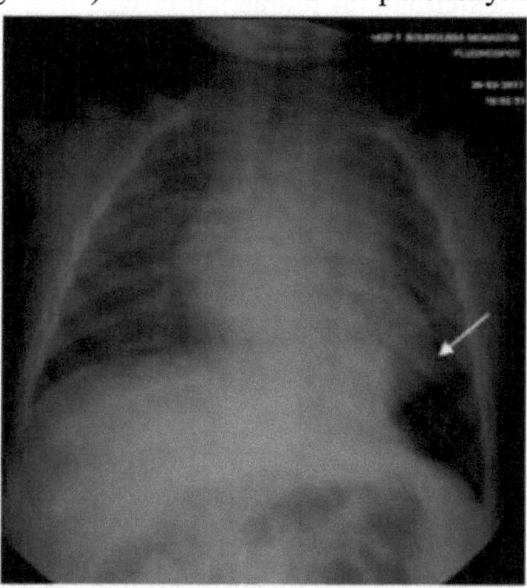

Fig.16: Front thoracic X-ray showing left lower parenchymal condensation (white arrow)

Trans-thoracic Doppler ultrasound confirmed the presence of an artery originating from the thoracic aorta and heading towards the sequestration.

A thoracic CT scan (figure 17) performed at the age of 2 months revealed a parenchymal condensation fed by an arterial branch originating from the descending thoracic aorta and drained by a branch of the left inferior pulmonary vein. This was consistent with intra-lobar pulmonary sequestration.

Given the high anaesthetic risk presented by the patient, it was decided to operate on his congenital heart disease and to schedule cold surgery for his bronchopulmonary malformation.

At the age of 5 months, he underwent percutaneous pulmonary valvuloplasty.

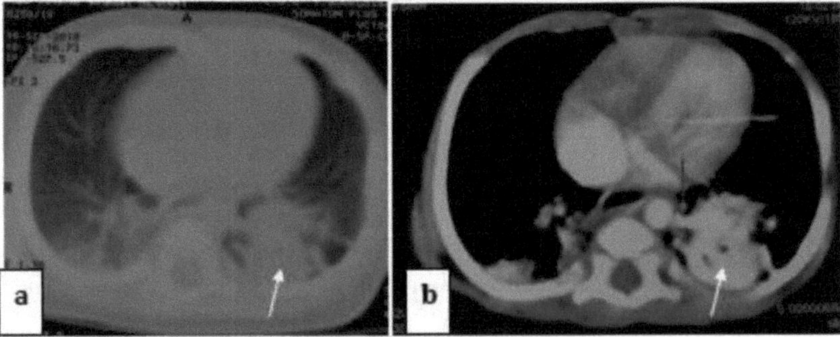

Fig.17(a,b): Axial section thoracic CT in parenchymal (a) and mediastinal (b) windows showing postëro-basal left parenchymal condensation (white arrows) with visualization of the feeder vessel originating from the left lateral wall of the thoracic aorta (red arrow).

At the age of 9 months, the infant underwent surgery for his bronchopulmonary malformation. A left posterolateral thoracotomy was performed. Intraoperative exploration revealed a left inferior lobar rosatre formation, vascularised by three systemic arteries originating from the thoracic aorta. Venous blood from this lung formation was drained by the left inferior pulmonary vein (Figure 18). This appearance was suggestive of intra-lobar pulmonary sequestration. After vascular ligation, a left inferior lobectomy was performed to remove the sequestration and a chest tube N°20 was inserted.

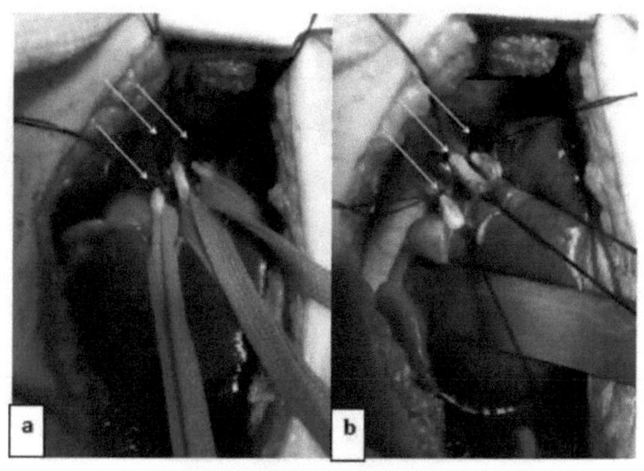

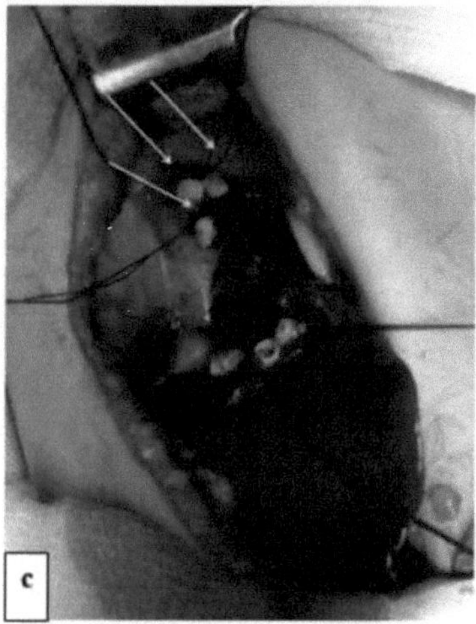

Fig.18(a,b,c): Intraoperative appearance of a left inferior lobar sequestration fed by three sytemic arteries from the thoracic aorta (white arrows).

Macroscopic examination (Figure 19) showed a specimen measuring 9cm in height and 3.7cm in thickness. On sectioning, the parenchyma showed a haemorrhagic appearance in the peripheral part of the specimen.

was straightforward. The follow-up chest X-ray showed good lung expansion (figure 24). The follow-up was 7 years.

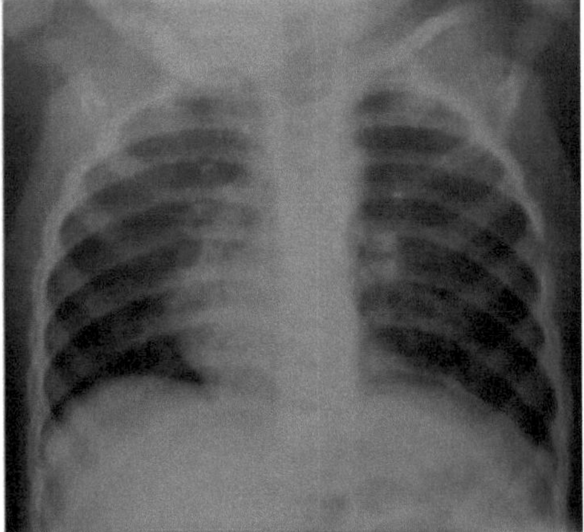

Fig.24: Front chest X-ray showing good post-opёratory left lung expansion.

Comment 11:

A 22-month-old male infant (B.A) from a normal pregnancy presented with bronchopneumonia at 9 months, treated with antibiotics. The fever subsided and respiratory signs improved. Radiological examination revealed persistent basi-thoracic opacity on the left (Figure 25).

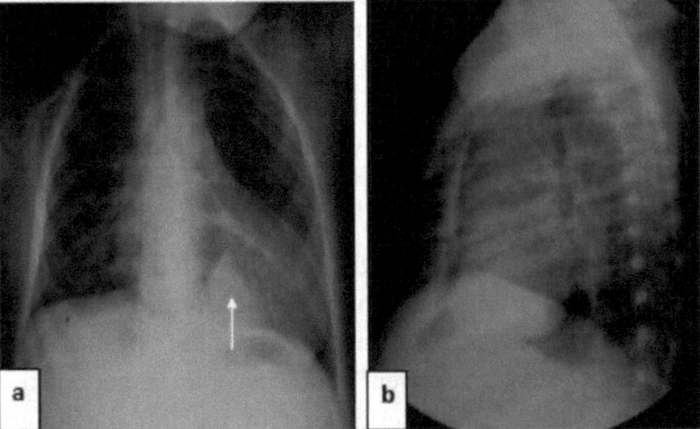

Fig.25: Front (a) and side (b) chest X-ray showing a left basi- thoracic opacйё (white arrow).

A thoracic CT and MRI scan ordered at a distance from the infectious episode concluded that the appearance was suggestive of a left post-basal pulmonary sequestration, showing a left paravertebral tissue mass measuring 60x40x30mm, fed by systёmic vessels (Figure 26,27).

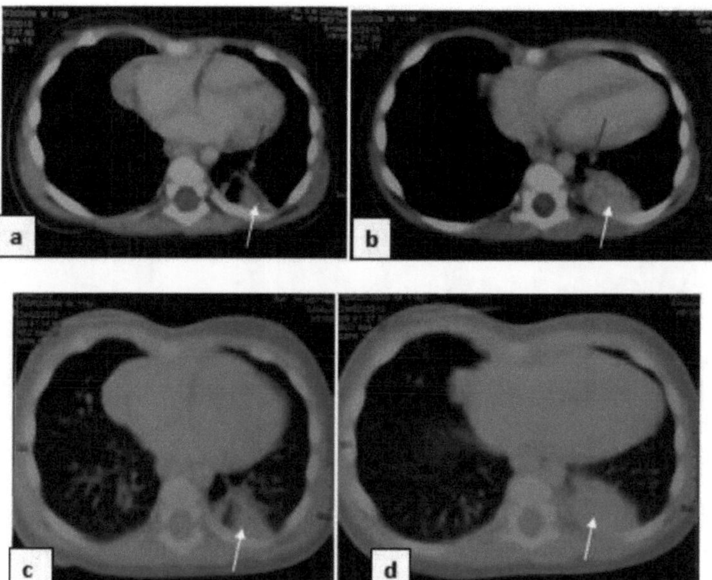

Fig.26(a,b,c,d): Chest CT scan in axial sections, mediastinal window (a,b) and parenchymal window (c,d) showing a left paravertebral tissue mass (white arrows) fed by systëmic vessels (red arrows).

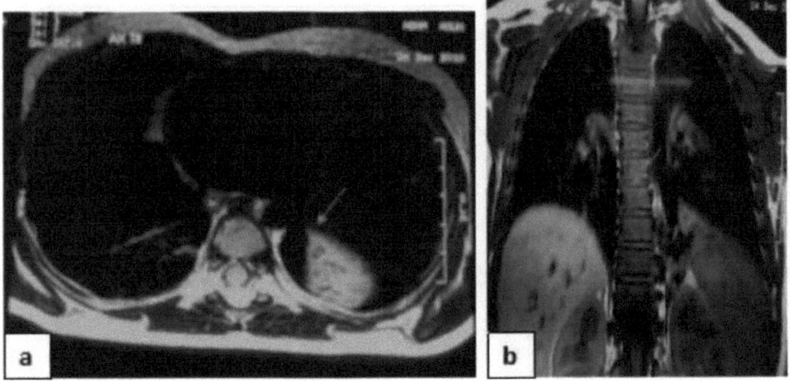

Fig.27(a,b): Axial T2-weighted MRI of the thorax (a) and coronal T2-weighted MRI (b). T1 (b) showing extra-lobar sequestration (green arrows)

The decision was made to operate on the patient. Exploration by thoracoscopy revealed a left extra-lobar pulmonary sequestration, vascularised by four vessels: two arteries and two veins (Figure 28). These vessels were ligated with clips, followed by resection of the sequestration and its exteriorisation through the trocar orifice (Figure 29).

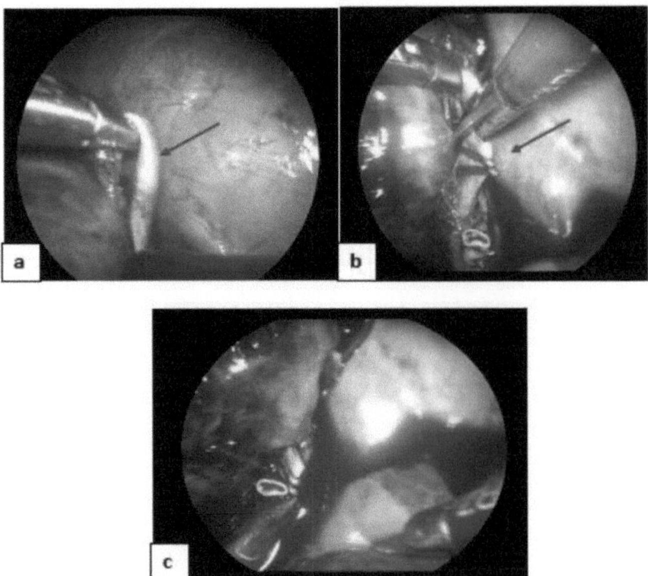

Fig 28(a,b,c): Intraoperative aspect showing riiemostasis by clip of the feeding vessels vessels

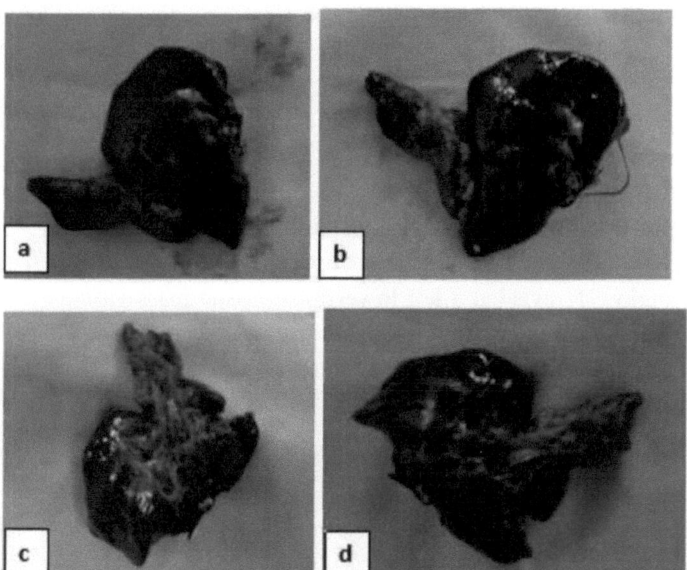

Fig.29(a,b,c,d): Intraoperative aspect of extra-lobar sequestration

On pathological examination, the specimen was heterogeneous and hemorrhagic, measuring 50x40x25mm, with pus and mucus in the lumina of the bronchi and bronchioles.

The post-operative course was straightforward, with removal of the chest tube on D3 post-operatively. The chest X-ray on discharge showed good lung expansion (Figure 30). The follow-up was 11 years.

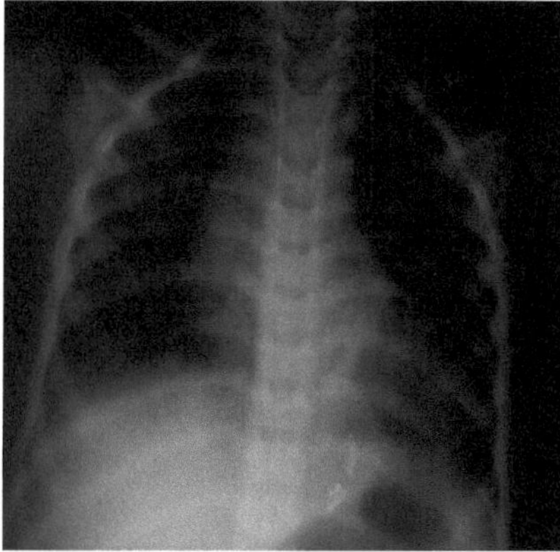

Fig.30: Front thoracic X-ray showing good post-operative expansion of the left lung with no significant parenchymal condensation.

Comment 12:

Female infant (K.I), 1 month old, from a normal pregnancy, carried to term.
Obstetric ultrasound at 20 weeks' gestation showed a hyperechogenic appearance of the lower lobe of the left lung with the presence of two aberrant systemic vessels. Exploration of the intra-abdominal viscera and the heart was normal.
Delivery was by cesarean section for fatal macrosomia and scarred uterus. At birth, she presented with moderate neonatal respiratory distress.
The chest X-ray showed left paracardiac opacity.
Thoracic angio-CT revealed a left lower lobar tissue mass vascularised by two systemic arteries arising from the thoracic aorta, strongly suggesting the diagnosis of pulmonary sequestration (figure 31).

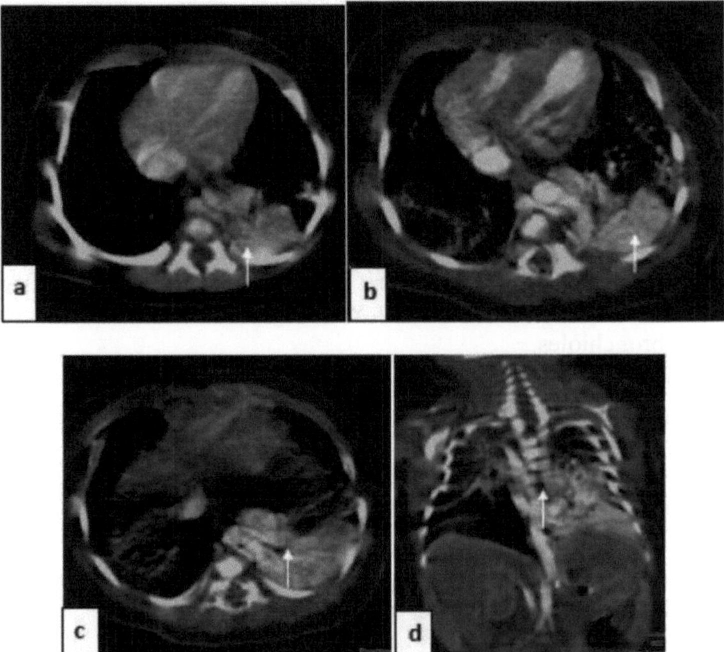

Fig.31(a,b,c,d): Thoracic CT angiography, in the mëdiastinal window, in axial (a, b, c) and coronal (d) sections showing the appearance of left infëterior extra-lobar sequestration (white arrows).

A left thoracoscopy was performed. Intraoperative exploration revealed a left posterolateral pulmonary formation adjacent to the lower lobe and separated from it by a pleura. This formation, which corresponded to the extra-lobar sequestration, was vascularised by four vessels: two arteries and two veins. After coagulation and vascular sectioning using an ultrascissor, the sequestration was exercized and then exteriorised through the trocar orifice (Figure 32).

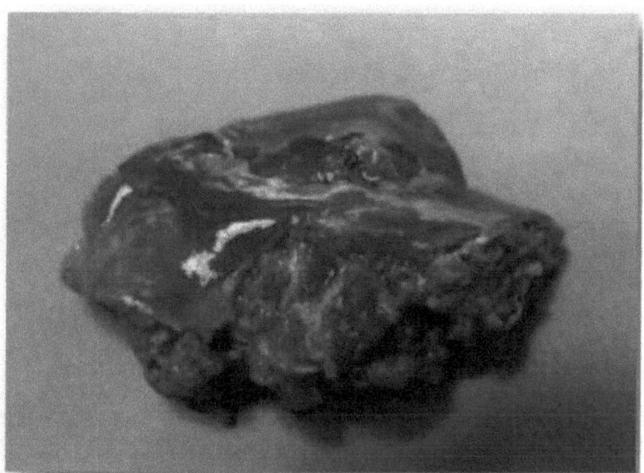

Fig.32: Surgical section of an MS

Histological examination showed lung tissue rich in bronchiolar structures and arterial-type vessels.

The post-operative course was straightforward. The drain was removed on day 2 post-operatively. The child was handed over to his parents at 9 days post-operatively. He did not present any respiratory signs. The follow-up was 9 years.

Comment 13:

NRS (K.H), 15 months old, female, was born at term by vaginal delivery, with antecedents of an episode of bronchoalveolitis treated in hospital with a good clinical course. On examination, lung auscultation showed a decrease in left-sided vesicular murmurs.

A chest X-ray was ordered and showed a digestive clara projecting into the left lung field. A thoracic computed tomography (CT) scan showed an ascension of the gastric greater curvature and the spleen in the left intra-thoracic region. The infant underwent thoracoscopic surgery. Intraoperative exploration revealed a left diaphragmatic hernia with the presence of the spleen and part of the stomach intra-thoracically. In addition, there was a pinkish, extra-lobar pulmonary malformation adherent to the hernia sac. The decision was to reduce the hernia contents, close the diaphragmatic defect and then excise and exteriorise the hernia sac, taking the pulmonary malformation with it after ligation of the systemic artery.

Histologically, the sample consisted of lung tissue, formed by cavities resembling bronchioles lined with respiratory-type epithelium. These cavities were separated from one another by sparse connective tissue, with no alveolar structures in between. This appearance was very reminiscent of the microscopic appearance of adenomatoid cystic malformation of the lung type 2. However, this malformed lung tissue was extra-lobar. It therefore corresponded to extra-lobar pulmonary sequestration.

The post-operative course was straightforward, with no respiratory symptoms. The follow-up chest X-ray showed good lung expansion. The follow-up was 16 years.

Comment 14:

A 5-year-old girl (S.A) with no notable pathological antecedents was admitted to hospital with a productive cough evolving in a febrile setting.

Clinical examination revealed a deterioration in general condition, with polypnoea and crepitus rales in the right lung base.

The chest X-ray showed a well-limited opacity occupying the upper two-thirds of the right pulmonary hemi-chamber with the presence of a hydro-aeric level (figure 33). The diagnosis of hydatid cyst of the emesis lung was the most likely. Abdominal ultrasound revealed no hydatid localization in the liver and hydatid serology was not performed.

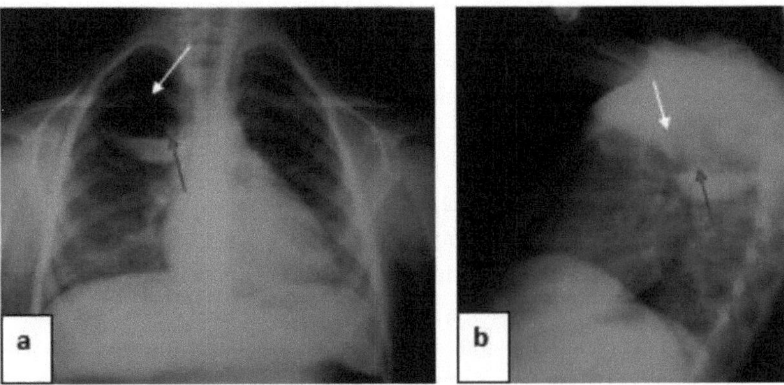

Fig.33(a,b): Chest X-ray, front (a) and side (b), showing well-limited excised opacity of the right hemi-lung field (white arrows) with the presence of a hydro-aeric level (red arrows).

A thoracic CT scan was ordered, which showed a large cystic formation in the right upper lobe with a hydro-aerobic content (Figure 34).

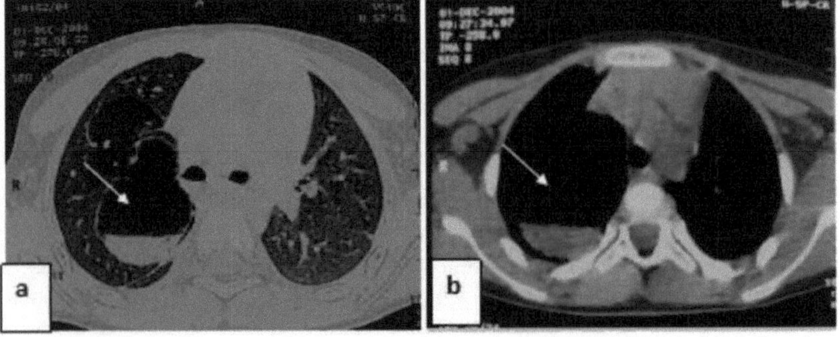

Fig.34(a,b): Chest CT scan with parenchymal (a) and mediastinal (b) windows showing a right upper lobar cystic formation with hydroaerobic content (white arrow).

The child underwent right posterolateral thoracotomy. Investigation revealed a mediastinal cystic mass that did not adhere to the lung parenchyma but did adhere to the trachea. Dissection of the adhesions revealed the presence of a feeder vessel for the mass. After ligation of this vessel, complete exeresis of the mass was performed. Its appearance was reminiscent of a bronchogenic cyst (Figure 35).

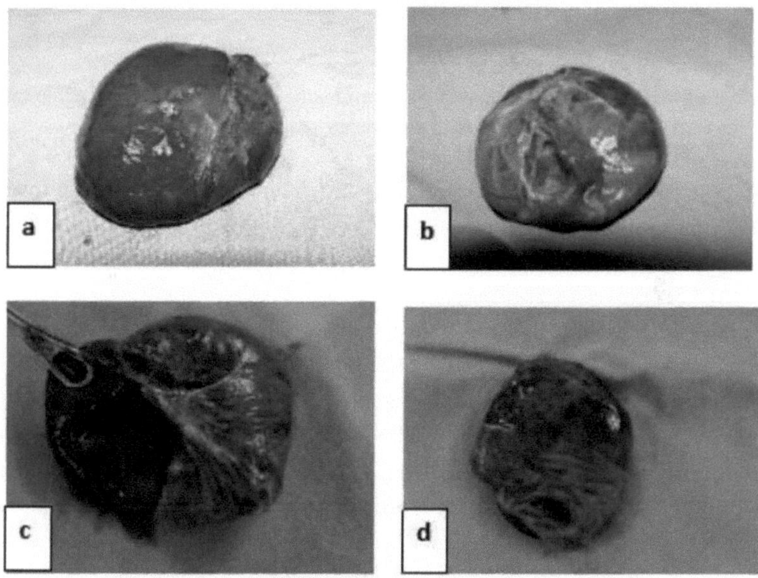

Fig.35(a,b,c,d): Operating part

Histological examination showed basophilic cubic epithelium over a sparsely cellular connective tissue. This connective tissue contained bronchial-type seromucosal acinar glands. On another section, structures reminiscent of pulmonary alveoli were associated.

This confirmed the diagnosis of a bronchogenic cyst developed in an extra-lobar pulmonary sequestration (figure 36).

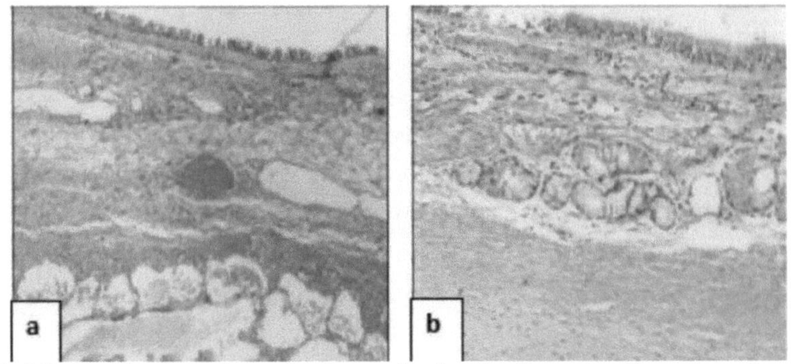

Fig.36(a,b): Histological examination confirming the diagnosis of bronchogenic cyst associated with pulmonary sequestration

The post-operative course was straightforward. The chest tube was removed at 3 days post-operatively. The follow-up chest X-ray showed no abnormalities. The follow-up was 16 years.

Comment 15:

A 3-month-old female infant (C.M) was born at term by Caesarean section to a primigravida primiparous mother. The pregnancy progressed normally. An antenatal ultrasound and MRI scan revealed a cystic lung mass. At birth, the newborn was asymptomatic and the physical examination was without abnormalities. A chest X-ray showed a clear, well-limited, rounded image occupying the upper left pulmonary hemichampus (Figure 37).

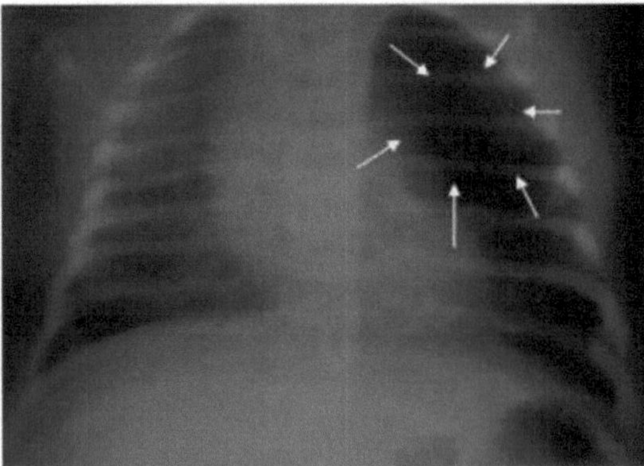

Fig.37: Front thoracic X-ray showing a well-limited left apical cleft (white arrows).

Thoracic computed tomography (CT) showed a left apico-dorsal cystic mass measuring 40x40x30mm, mono-locular, with a thin wall and containing a hydro-aerobic level. This cystic mass had no obvious systemic arterial vascularisation.

The infant was operated on at the age of 3 months via a left posterolateral thoracotomy. Intraoperative exploration revealed a mediastino-pulmonary cystic formation 80 x 5mm in diameter in contact with the left upper lobe and enclosing a tongue of lung parenchyma. Dissection of this cyst revealed arterial vascularisation provided by a 3mm diameter vessel draining into the aorta and venous vascularisation draining into the pulmonary system. A sequestrectomy was performed and a chest tube was inserted. Macroscopic examination showed a thin-walled, brownish cyst 50mm in diameter. Histological examination was in favour of a bronchogenic cyst developed in an extra-lobar pulmonary sequestration. The post-operative course was straightforward, with the drain removed at 3 days post-operatively. The chest X-ray showed good post-operative lung expansion (Figure 38). The follow-up was 3 years.

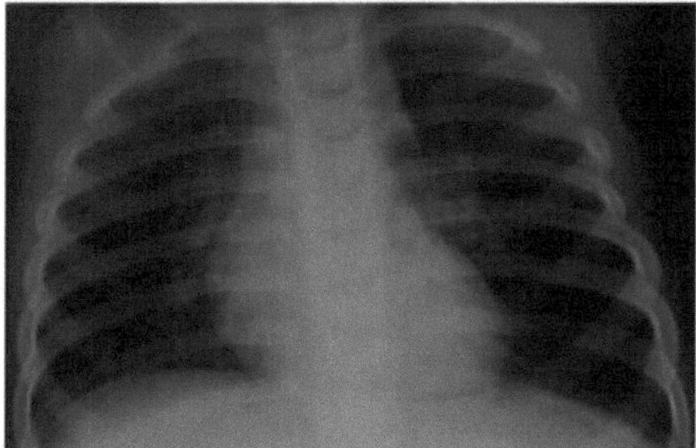

Fig.38: Front chest X-ray taken 1 year post-operatively showing good expansion of the left lung.

Comment 16:

Male infant (B.A), 10 months old, from a normal pregnancy, carried to term, by a primigravida primiparous mother.

Obstetric ultrasound at 18 weeks' gestation showed multiple cystic lesions in the left basal lung.

The delivery was carried out to term, vaginally, without incident. The clinical examination at birth was without anomalies. However, at the age of 1 month, he developed mild dyspnoea with a cough evolving in a context of apyrexia. The chest X-ray showed left basal clefts projecting onto the cardiac silhouette (Figure 39).

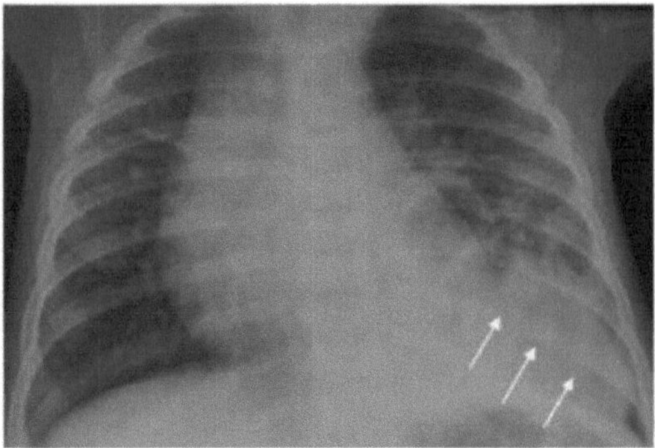

Fig.39: Front chest X-ray showing left basal condensation (white arrows)

Thoracic angioscan showed partial condensation of the left lower lobe with cystic images of variable size, vascularised by three vessels arising directly from the thoracic aorta and abnormal venous return from the azygos system (Figure 40,41). This was strongly suggestive of intra-lobar pulmonary sequestration.

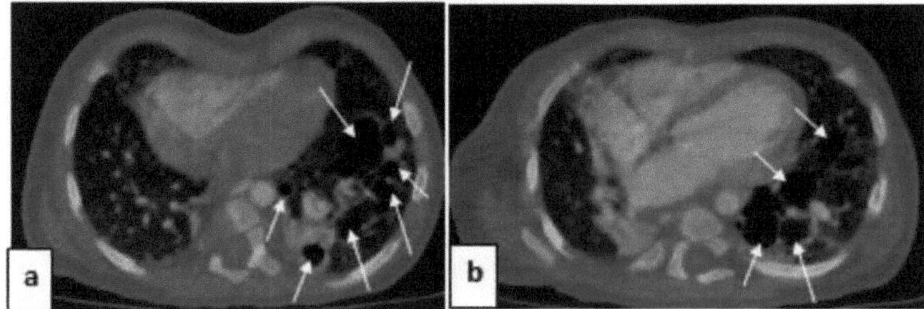

Fig.40(a,b): Chest CT angiography with parenchymal window showing cystic images of variable size in the left lower lobe (white arrows).

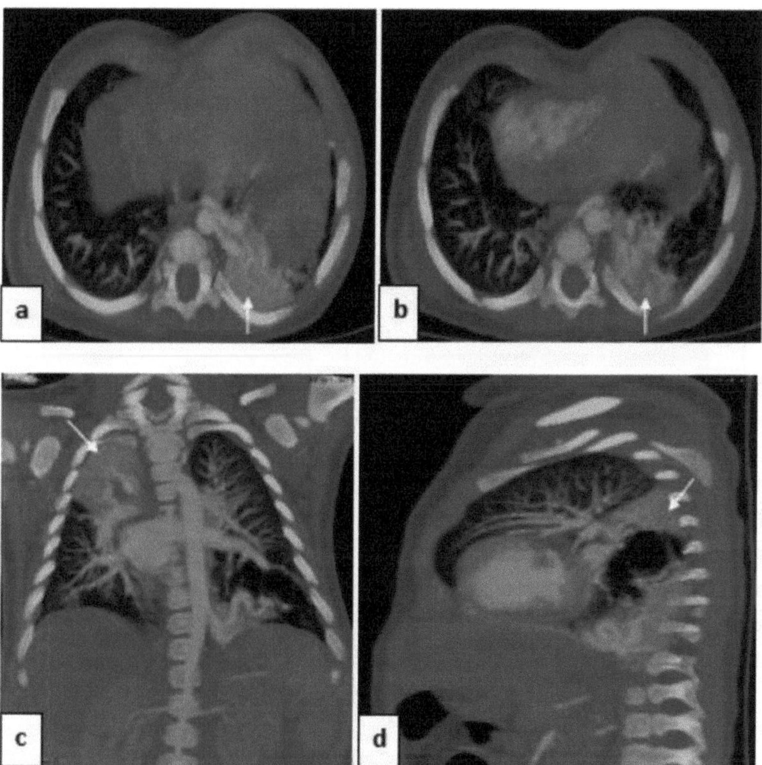

Fig.41(a,b,c,d): Thoracic CT angiography in axial (a,b), coronal (c) and sagittal (d) sections with MIP (maximum intensity projection) showing the origin of the systëmic vessels from the thoracic aorta (a,b) (red arrows) diverting towards the sëquestration (white arrows) with abnormal venous return at the level of the azygos system (c,d).

The infant was operated on via a left posterolateral thoracotomy. After release of adhesions, intraoperative exploration revealed a left lower lobe, which was the site of several cystic formations at the level of the basal pyramid with the presence of four systemic vessels approximately 3 cm above the diaphragm, arising from the thoracic aorta. Venous drainage was provided by a large 8mm vein leading to the anterior mediastinum. After vascular ligation, a left inferior lobectomy was performed (Figure 42).

The average age of the patients was 18.5 months, with extremes ranging from 1 day to 10 years.

1.4. Breakdown by gender

The breakdown by gender was as follows:

Seven boys and 9 girls, giving a sex ratio of 7/9 (0.77).

It was 4/8 (0.5) for SEL and 3 for SIL (Figure 45).

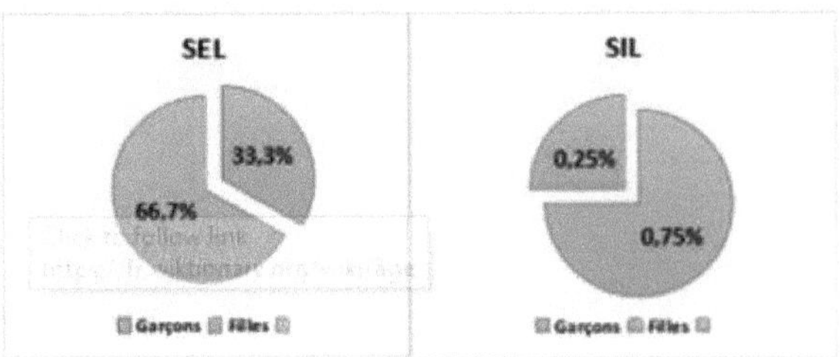

Fig.45: Breakdown of patients by sex

2. CLINICAL STUDY

2. 1. Background

> **Family:**

Questioning revealed no family history of congenital malformations, particularly bronchopulmonary.

> **Staff:**

Delivery was at term in 15 of 16 cases (93.75%), by vaginal delivery in 10 of 16 cases (62.5%) and by cesarean section in 6 of 16 cases (37.5%).

2.2 Circumstances of discovery

2.2.1 Antenatal diagnosis

Antenatal ultrasound was accurate in 8 children (8/16) (50%). The mean age of antenatal diagnosis was 21 days' gestation, with extremes ranging from 16 to 30 days' gestation. The lesion was unilateral in all cases. Two fetuses had pleural effusion with associated mediastinal deviation (cases 2, 4). No associated malformations were noted.

Freight MRI was performed in 4 patients (4/16) (25%). It strongly suspected the diagnosis of pulmonary sequestration in only one case (1/4). It also confirmed the presence of a bronchopulmonary malformation in the remaining cases.

No antenatal lung lesions showed spontaneous resolution or regression.

In the light of antenatal imaging data, the origin of pulmonary malformations was suggested, but an etiological diagnosis could not be made.

Additional post-natal tests are required to establish a positive diagnosis.

2. 2. 2 Post-natal revelation

Antenatal diagnosis was lacking in our series in 8 patients (8/16) (50%).

> **Immediate (neonatal)**

Three newborns (3/8) with antenatal diagnosis of MBP were symptomatic. The neonatal respiratory distress was severe, requiring mechanical ventilation in 2/3 cases (cases 2, 4) and moderate in 1/3 cases (case 12).

The severity of the clinical picture was associated with the presence of ultrasound signs of gravity during antenatal care (pleural effusion, mediastinal deviation) (cases 2, 4).

> **Late**

These were recurrent bronchiolitis in 3 cases /16 (cases n° 5, 6, 7) and febrile pneumonia in 4 cases /16 (cases n° 8, 11, 14, 16).

In addition, pulmonary sequestration was discovered incidentally during surgery for a hernia of the diaphragmatic dome in 3 out of 16 cases (cases 9, 10, 13).

2. 3. Physical examination

On inspection, polypnea was present in 11 cases/16 (68.7%), accompanied by signs of struggle in 7 out of 16 cases (43.7%).

On auscultation, tachycardia and reduced vesicular murmurs in the homolateral hemithorax were found in 6/16 cases (37.5%).

Snoring rales were noted in 3 cases /16 (18.7%), crepitating rales in 1 case /16 and auscultatory silence in 4 cases /16 (25%).

Finally, fever was observed in 6 out of 16 cases (37.5%).

The physical examination was normal in 5 out of 16 cases (31.2%).

3. 3. Associated malformations

Clinical examination revealed a heart murmur in only one patient, related to valvular pulmonary narrowing (case 7). However, cardiac ultrasound was performed in only 3 of the 16 cases.

In the light of the clinical data, the malformative origin was confirmed by antenatal diagnosis and suggested for the other 8 children. The etiology of the malformation was investigated by means of additional tests.

4. FURTHER TESTS

4.1.Prenatal imaging

4.1.1. Prenatal ultrasound

Morphological ultrasound performed in the second trimester of pregnancy strongly suspected the diagnosis of pulmonary sequestration in 2/8 cases, showing :

- A hyperechogenic mass in the left hemithorax with the presence of a systemic vessel (case 7);
- A hyperechogenic appearance of the lower lobe of the left lung with the

presence of two aberrant systemic vessels originating from the thoracic aorta (case 12);

In the remaining cases (6/8), where the systemic vessel was not visualised, ultrasound was objective:

- A hyperechogenic appearance of the left lower lobe in 2 cases (12.5%) (cases 1, 16);
- A hyperechogenic appearance of the right lower lobe in one case (case 4);
- A hyperechogenic appearance of the upper left lobe in one case (case 15).
- A hyperechogenic retro-cardiac mass anterior to and in contact with the aorta (case 3).
- Large pleural effusion with mediastinal deviation in 2 cases (12.5%) (cases 2, 4).

However, these images are not specific to pulmonary sequestration.

4.1.2. Fatal MRI

Fetal MRI was performed in 4 patients (4/16) (50%). It confirmed the ultrasound findings in these patients, demonstrating a T1 hyposignal, T2 hypersignal thoracic lung parenchymal mass. It also confirmed the presence of an aberrant systemic vessel in one case (1/4) (case 7).

Fatal MRI was performed in 4 patients, and the diagnosis of pulmonary sequestration was made in only one case.

4.2.Post-natal imaging

3.2.1 Standard chest X-ray

All our patients had a frontal chest X-ray. This investigation was carried out from birth in the case of antenatal diagnosis, and from the onset of the first symptoms in the other patients.

She has an objective:

- Parenchymal opacity in 4 cases /16, of postero-basal left siege in one case /4 (case n° 11) and occupying the right pulmonary hemichamp in 3 cases /4 (case n° 5,8,14).

This opacity was associated with a hydro-aeric level in one case/4 (case 5).

- Left paracardiac opacity in 2 out of 16 cases (cases 6, 12).

- Posterior opacity, retro-cardiac in 1/16 cases (case 3).

- Lung parenchymal condensation in 3 cases/16 (cases 1,7,16) associated with compensatory contralateral hypertrophy in two patients (2/3).

- A well-limited left apical cleft in 1 case/16 (case n° 15).

- Intra-thoracic digestive tracts, suggestive of herniation of the left diaphragmatic dome in 3 cases/16 (cases 9, 10, 13).

- Reflux of the mediastinum was found in 9 cases/16 (cases n° 2,4,5,7,9,10,11,13).

In addition, in 2 patients (2/16), the chest X-ray showed a large pleural effusion. After pleural drainage, the diagnosis of bronchopulmonary malformation was suspected, in the absence of clinical improvement (cases 2, 4).

In total, the chest X-ray allowed the diagnosis of herniation of the left diaphragmatic cupola to be retained in 3 cases out of 16 (18.75%). In the remaining cases (13/16) (81.25%), a pulmonary anomaly was suspected because of the persistence of the radiological anomaly. Further investigations were therefore necessary.

3.2.2 Transthoracic Doppler ultrasound

In our series, it was performed in 3 patients (3/16) (18.75%). In only one patient (1/3) (case 7) was the diagnosis of pulmonary sequestration confirmed by identification of a systemic artery arising from the thoracic aorta and leading to the sequestration.

3.2.3 Thoracic CT angiography

A thoracic CT scan with contrast injection was carried out in all our patients and showed :

- Pulmonary parenchymal condensation fed by systemic arterial branches in 4 cases/16 (25%) (cases 1, 4, 7, 16);

- Thin-walled pulmonary cystic formations with air content in 5 of 16 cases (31.25%) (cases 5, 6, 8, 14, 15).

- A mediastinal tissue mass supplied by an artery from the aorta in 3 patients (3/16) (18.75%) (cases N° 3, 11, 12).

- Intra-thoracic digestive bleeding in 3 patients (3/16) (18.75%) (cases N° 9, 10, 13).

- A multi-cloisonne pleural effusion without finding any underlying cause or associated malformation, in only one case out of 16 (case N° 2).

3.2.4 Thoracic MRI angiography

A thoracic MRI scan after birth was carried out in only one case (case 11), in whom exploration by X-ray and thoracic CT scan had suspected the diagnosis of pulmonary sequestration. It showed a left posterobasal lung parenchymal condensation with an iso T1 signal, moderate T2 hypersignal and intense enhancement after injection of gadolinium. Within this mass, serpiginous vascular structures originating from the aorta and others joining the intra- and peri-spinal venous plexus were identified.

4.3.Location

The topography of the lesions selected on completion of the additional examinations is shown in **Table II.**

Location	Number of cases	Percentage (%)
Left side	12	75
Right-hand dimension	4	25
TOTAL	16	100

Table II: Distribution of patients according to MS location

3.4 Diagnostic imaging

On the basis of imaging data, the diagnosis of pulmonary sequestration was made in 7 of 16 cases (43.75%). It was associated with MAKP in 2/7 cases (12.5%). The other diagnoses were an isolated MAKP in 2 cases/16 (12.5%), a hydatid cyst of the lung in one case/16, a bronchogenic cyst or a pleuropericardial cyst or an esophageal duplication in one case/16, a MAKP associated with a bronchogenic cyst in one case/16 and a recurrent pleural effusion of undetermined etiology in a single patient (1/16). The diagnosis of herniation of the left diaphragmatic dome without any other associated malformation was accepted in 3 patients (3/16) (18.75%).

3.5 Malformation assessment

Cardiac ultrasound in 3 children (3/16) (cases 4, 7, 12) was pathological in 2/3 cases (4, 7), revealing atrial septal defect in one case (4) and pulmonary valvular narrowing in one case (7).

All in all:

The diagnosis of pulmonary sequestration was initially evoked by the clinical-radiological picture in only 7 of 16 cases (43.75%).

The main diagnostic feature was the visualization of an aberrant systemic artery.

3. SURGICAL TREATMENT

4.1.Pre-natal treatment

Two fetuses (12.5%) had a large pleural effusion with mediastinal deviation on antenatal ultrasound but were not treated antenatally (cases 2,4).

4.2.Post-natal treatment

All 16 patients had respiratory symptoms that led to the decision to undergo surgery.

Surgery was planned for 13 children (13/16). The remaining 3 cases underwent emergency surgery for acute respiratory distress secondary to herniation of the diaphragmatic dome.

4.2.1 Preparing the patient

> **Generale**

It was based on a request for a blood count, a hemostasis test and an iso-group iso-rhesus phenotype blood reserve outside the emergency department.

> **Respiratory**

It was based on respiratory kinesitherapy.

4.2.2 Anaesthesia

General anaesthesia was administered via orotracheal intubation.
Hemodynamic and respiratory monitoring is essential.
Antibiotic prophylaxis with betalactam was systematic.
Intraoperative analgesia was provided by morphine spinal anaesthesia and infiltration of the surgical scar.

4.2.3 Approach route

> **Posterolateral thoracotomy at the level of the 5 EIC^{eme}**

It was performed on 7 patients (7/16) (43.75%) (cases 4, 5, 7, 8, 14, 15, 16).
Patients were positioned in the lateral decubitus position, with the homolateral upper limb elevated and a sub-costal log in place.

> **Median laparotomy**

It was performed on a single patient with a left diaphragmatic hernia associated with a volvulus of the stomach (case 9).

> **Thoracoscopy**

This was the approach in 8 patients (8/16) (50%) (cases 1, 2, 3, 6, 10, 11, 12, 13). The patients were positioned in lateral decubitus on the side opposite the lesion, with a subcutaneous block in place.
A first 5mm optical trocar was inserted below the scapula, at the intersection between the anterior axillary line and the 5eme intercostal space. A pneumothorax was created by insufflation of CO2 (pressure of 8 millimetres of mercury) to provide a working space. Two or three 5 mm operating trocars were placed in triangulation and behind the axillary line.
conversion was 37.5% (3 cases/8) (cases 1, 2, 6).
This thoracoscopic approach enabled the bronchopulmonary malformation to be treated in 31.25% of cases (5 cases/16) (cases 3, 10, 11, 12, 13).
The reasons for conversion were the occurrence of uncontrollable bleeding in one case (case 1) and dissection difficulties in the remaining 2 cases (cases 2, 6).

4.2.4 Intraoperative findings

> **Type:**

Surgical exploration revealed a parenchymal formation independent of the lung and surrounded by its own pleura in 12 of 16 cases (75%). This appearance was suggestive of extra-lobar sequestration. In the remaining 4 cases (25%), an area of dystrophy contrasted with normal adjacent parenchyma, suggestive of intra-lobar sequestration.

> **Topography:**

The left side was affected in 12 of 16 cases (75%). Sequestration occurred on the right side in 4 of 16 cases (25%).

In all cases, there was agreement between the radiological topographical distribution adopted in the pre-operative phase and that observed in the peri-operative phase.

> **Arterial contribution:**

- **SEL :** The origin of the systemic artery was:
- Thoracic aorta in 3 cases/12 (25%) (cases 4,12,15).
- Abdominal aorta in 2 cases/12 (16.66%) (cases 2, 11).
- Celiac trunk in 1 case/12 (case 3).
- Not specified in the operative report: 6 cases/12 (50%) (cases 5,6,9,10,13,14).

> **SIL :** The origin of the systemic artery was:

> Thoracic aorta in 3 cases/4 (75%) (cases 1, 7, 16).

> Abdominal aorta in 1 case/4 (case 8).

> **Number of systemic arteries:**

On average 1 to 2 systemic arteries, with extremes ranging from 1 to 4, and 81.25% of cases were vascularised by a single systemic artery.

> **Diameter:**

The average diameter of the systemic arteries was 3 mm, with extremes ranging from 0.5 to 6 mm.

> **Venous return:**

It was provided by the pulmonary venous system in 3 cases/4 of SIL and by the azygos system in one case.

For SELs, it was provided by the azygos system in 3 cases out of 16.

In the remaining cases, venous return was not specified.

> **Surgical procedure**

The surgical procedure consisted of lobectomy in 5 patients (5/16) (31.25%) and sequestrectomy in 11 patients (11/16) (68.75%). In the case of herniation of the diaphragmatic dome (3/16), we opted for reduction of the hernial contents and closure of the diaphragmatic defect. For gastric volvulus, stomach detorsion and gastropexy were performed.

4. Associated malformations (Table III):

	Hernia of the diaphragmatic dome	MAKP	Bronchogenic cyst	Congenital heart disease
SP	3 cases	4 cases	4 cases	2 cases

Table III: The different associated malformations present in our patients

5.ANATOMOPATHOLOGICAL EXAMINATION

Anatomopathological study of the resection specimen confirmed the diagnosis of sequestration in all cases, showing a sequestration consisting of several cavities with either a bronchial structure or a collagen wall covered with cylindrical or flattened epithelium.

From a vascular point of view, the artery was a systemic artery of the elastic type.

In total, pathological examination confirmed the diagnosis of SEL in 12 of 16 cases (75%) and SIL in 4 of 16 cases (25%).

6. POST-OPERATIONS

All the patients followed had a good outcome. Extubation was immediate on complete awakening of the patient in all cases. Preventive antibiotic therapy (Amoxicillin and clavulanic acid at a dose of 100 milligrams per kilogram) was continued for 3 to 5 days. The anterior chest tube was removed between 2eme and 3 ^{eme}post-operatively. In one patient, a 2eme posterior chest tube was inserted and removed between 5eme and 7eme days. The post-operative radiograph was satisfactory with good lung expansion. All patients benefited from post-operative physiotherapy and respiratory therapy. The average length of hospital stay was 7 days.

7.FOLLOW-UP

The patients operated on were followed up at the paediatric surgery and paediatrics outpatient clinic, with an average follow-up of 9 years.

Apart from a single case of recurrence of left diaphragmatic hernia (case 10), all our patients had a favourable clinical and radiological outcome, with disappearance of respiratory signs and radiological abnormalities.

None of our patients developed bronchopneumonia after the operation.

However, no respiratory function tests were carried out.
In addition, no orthopaedic sequelae, particularly of the spine, were encountered, with good staturo-ponderal development.

8. MORTALITY

No cases of death have been reported in our series.

DISCUSSION

I/ EPIDEMIOLOGICAL STUDY

1. Incidence and frequency

Pulmonary sequestration is a rare bronchopulmonary malformation. It accounts for 0.15 to 6.5% of lung malformations [2,4,5].
Its incidence is estimated at between 0.15 and 1.8%. It is probably underestimated, as the diagnosis may still be made in the adult population, in patients with or without symptoms [5,6].
Its prevalence is currently unknown. Advances in obstetric imaging techniques have increased the number of lung sequestrations diagnosed antenatally [5,6].
Intra-lobar sequestration is the most common, accounting for around 75% of cases in the literature [9,10,11,12,13]. The extra-lobar form is less common, accounting for 25% of cases [9,10,11,12,13].
In our series, sequestrations accounted for 8.3% of MBPs. Contrary to the literature, SELs were the most frequent (75%). Similarly, an American series published in 2015 found a clear predominance of SEL (62%) in children [14] (**Table IV**). This could be explained by the age of recruitment and the latency of LIS, which is often diagnosed in adolescence or adulthood [11,12,13,14].

2. Sex ratio

The authors unanimously agreed that SEL is predominantly male, with a sex ratio of 4:1. No pathogenic explanation was found to explain this male predominance.
For SIL, there is no gender predominance [15,16,17].
In our series, we noted a predominance of females in the extra-lobar type.

3. Location

MS occurs in 98% of cases in the lower lobes [2,14,16].
Seventy-five per cent of SELs arise between the diaphragm and the lower lobe and in 80% of cases on the left, whereas SILs arise in the posterobasal region of the lower lobe without a predominance of sides [16]. Localisation in the middle lobe is very rare, as is localisation in the upper lobe. Bilateral involvement is exceptional [2]. Our data are consistent with the literature.
Table IV compares the main series of pulmonary sequestration described in the literature.

Study	Number	Average age	Type	Gender	Country

	of cases	([a]n)			
Khen-Dunlop et al.,2018 [18]	99	<1	SIL 65 SEL 35%	M: 62% F: 38%	France
Tashtouch and all.,2015 [14]	8	<2	SIL 38% SEL 62	M: 52% F: 48%	United States
Ou et al.,2014 [19]	30	4,3	SIL 77% SEL 23	M: 40% F: 60%	China
Gezer et al., 2007	6	23,3	SIL 70% SEL 30%	M: 63% F: 37%	Turkey
[20]					
Van Raemdon ck et al., 2001 [21]	13	3	SIL 62 SEL 38%	M: 64% F: 36%	Belgium
Halkic et al, 1998 [22]	22 4	<1	SIL 73% SEL 27%	M: 62% F: 38%	Switzerland

Table IV: Comparative study of the main series of pulmonary sequestration described in the literature

4. Embryology

The development of pulmonary sequestration occurs early in gestational life, between 5[eme] and 6[eme] weeks' gestation [4]. However, the embyological origin is still a subject of ongoing debate [14]. In 1861, Rokitansky introduced the first description of the disease. He stipulated that MS was due to a separation of a normally developed lung during organogenesis, the fraction theory [14]. Several other embryological malformative or acquired pathogenic hypotheses were subsequently described (**Table V**). In 1946, Pryce was the first to use the term "pulmonary sequestration" and classified the disease into intra-lobar and extra-lobar types [3]. The embryopathogenic explanation put forward by Pryce is mechanical, and is common to both extra- and intra-lobar sequestration [3]. Sequestration, in the bronchial sense, is thought to be the result of vascular traction exerted by the persistence of the systemic vessel, thus excluding this fragment of parenchyma from the normal tracheobronchial tree [14-22]. The chronology of this phenomenon would explain the difference between intra- and extra-lobar sequestration. If the malformation appears early, then sequestration will be intra-lobar. If the malformation appears after thoracic partitioning and pleural covering of the pericardium, then sequestration will be extra-lobar [14].

References	Theories
1861 Rokitansky	Separation of the normally developed lung
1878 Ruge	The malformation appears separate from the normal lung in the form of a third lung.
1946 Pryce	Traction theory: Vascular traction exerted by the persistence of the systemic vessel, thus excluding this fragment of parenchyma from the normal tracheobronchial tree.
1956 Smith	Theory of blood supply: Persistence of systemic vascularisation due to pulmonary arterial insufficiency
1958	No causal relationship between systemic artery and parenchyma
Boyden	non-functional lung
1959 Gebauer and Mason	Acquired anomaly theory: MS results from a relapsing localized infectious process
1967 Blesovsky	Failure of the signalling pathway and growth factors
1968 Gene et al.	Malformation congenital proentero-broncho-pulmonary (Congenital broncho pulmonary foregut malformation)
1968 Morscarella and Wylie	Intra-lobar sequestration is a collection of bronchial cysts associated with a systemic artery.
1984 Stocker and Malczak	Acquired theory: The systemic artery is a bronchial artery located in the triangular ligament.
1987 Clements and warne	Theory of malinosculation: Disruption of development normal bronchopulmonary

Table V: Theories described in the pathogenesis of pulmonary sequestration sequestration [14]

All in all, this history is relatively observational, based on operating embryos, then anatomical-radiological-surgical.

At present, the embryo-pathogenic explanation put forward by Pryce is the most widely adopted.

5. Classification

a- Typical forms (table VI)

These are both bronchial and arterial sequestrations (no communication with the healthy bronchial system and vascularisation by a systemic artery):

- **Intra-lobar sequestration**

The abnormal parenchyma is included in the lung parenchyma; they are contained in the same visceral vein [2].

The abnormal systemic artery arises from the descending thoracic aorta (75%) or abdominal aorta (20%) and the venous drainage is to a pulmonary vein [2]. According to Pryce, there are three types:

- type I: the only abnormality is vascularisation of an area of normal lung parenchyma by an artery of systemic origin;
- type II: the sequestrated lung parenchyma is formed from a normal bronchial bud. The abnormal artery supplies an area of sequestrated lung and part of the adjacent healthy lung;
- type III: the bronchial bud is normal but the supernumerary artery only vascularises the sequestrated lung [23].

- **Extra-lobar sequestration**

They have no connection with the normal lung and develop from a supernumerary bronchial bud. They have their own visceral pleural envelope. There is therefore a complete anatomical and physiological separation from the normal lung parenchyma. This form is associated with another malformation in 40% to 60% of cases, particularly a diaphragmatic hernia, pericardial dehiscence or bronchogenic cyst, unlike the intralobar forms [2].
The abnormal systemic artery arises from the terminal portion of the descending thoracic aorta (45%) or from the upper part of the abdominal aorta (32%) and enters the thorax through the triangular ligament [2]. In 15% of cases, the systemic artery has another origin: splenic, gastric, subclavian, diaphragmatic or intercostal [2]. Venous drainage is often systemic to the azygos, hemi-azygos or inferior vena cava [2].
For both types, the length of the artery varies according to its origin, as does its diameter, with an average of 6 mm [2].

CHARACTERISTICS DIFFERENTIALS	EXTRA-LOBAR	INTRA-LOBAR
Plevre	Surrounded by a clean pleural layer	Shares the visceral layer with the lung
Position	Postero-basal segment above or below the diaphragm	Postero-basal segment near the midline
Seat	90% left	60% left
Vascularisation	Arterial systemic Pulmonary artery	From the aorta to the diaphragm
Size of the systemic	Small artery	Large artery

vessel		
Drainage vein	Azygos or door system	Pulmonary vein rarely azygos
Communication with the digestive tract	Frequente	Plus, rare
Associated anomalies	Slow and low	Rare
Symptomatology	Early	Latent

Table VI: Classification of pulmonary sequestration [24].

b- Atypical forms:

Individualisation remains useful, as these are rare but sometimes very complex forms, associating sequestration with vascular or digestive malformations. The transition from SIL to SEL can be difficult to determine. Vascular anomalies are variable: abnormal venous return, either in the lungs outside the left atrium, or in the inferior vena cava. This may include scimitar syndrome, abnormal venous return in the inferior vena cava, with its typical radiological appearance [21].

In our series, the atypical form was not observed.

11- CLINICAL STUDY

1. Circumstances of discovery

1.1.Antenatal discovery

MS may be discovered prenatally, but requires referral to a specialist centre [25,26].

Among 21 antenatal MBPs, Lecomte reported only 2 cases of MS [27]. Similarly, Truit found only 2 cases among 35 antenatal MBPs [28].

However, in a French series published in 2018, the authors collected 99 paediatric cases of pulmonary sequestration, 86 of which were diagnosed antenatally [18].

In our series, MS was investigated in 8 antenatal patients, and was strongly suspected in 2 cases, a result which is close to previous series.

In its typical form, pulmonary sequestration appears as a homogenous triangular mass on the left posterobasal, hyperechogenic on ultrasound and hyperintense on MRI. The diagnosis is made with certainty by demonstration of the systemic feeder artery on MRI, which can easily be done by an experienced operator, or more simply by Doppler ultrasound. More rarely, in mixed forms (MAKP plus sequestration), associated cystic images may be seen, but it is the vascularisation of systemic origin that allows the diagnosis to be made [26].

Advances in antenatal imaging can improve the circumstances in which MS is discovered, but this requires advice from a specialist centre and collaboration between obstetricians, neonatologists, radiologists and

paediatric surgeons.

1.2.Post-natal discovery

1.2.1. In the neonatal period

The discovery of MS during the neonatal period is rare (25%) [29,30]. It is often asymptomatic, but may present as neonatal respiratory distress, especially in extra-lobar sequestration [30]. Pleural effusion or deviation of the mediastinum may also be observed and may even worsen until the appearance of hydrops [26].

In certain situations, the clinical symptomatology may be dominated by a picture of congestive heart failure due to a major shunt [31]. Khen-Dunlop found that in 86 newborns with antenatal diagnosis of MS, only 14% were symptomatic at birth [18].

In our series, neonatal respiratory distress was observed in 3 patients (18.75%), with mechanical ventilation in 2 cases. Two newborns required pleural drainage for profuse pleurisy.

1.2.2. After the neonatal period

Pulmonary sequestration is sometimes characterised by its clinical latency. When they become symptomatic, symptoms usually begin within the first two years. In a series of 99 sequestrations, Khen-Dunlop found that the mean age at diagnosis of symptomatic forms was 8 months [18].

The extra-lobar type manifests itself early, often in the first few months of life, with repeated lung infections or malaria. It is sometimes asymptomatic and may be discovered radiologically [14].

Intra-lobar sequestration is often diagnosed later. Repeated lung infections are the most common presenting sign [2,14]. Rarely, MS may be revealed by episodes of hemoptysis, hemothorax or heart failure [30]. Hemoptysis is due to the rupture of aneurysmal formations developed at the expense of the aberrant vessel [32].

In our series, 3 infants presented with acute bronchiolitis and 4 with febrile pneumonitis. In addition, 3 patients in our series underwent surgery for herniation of the diaphragmatic dome with incidental intraoperative discovery of MS.

III ADDITIONAL TESTS

1. Chest X-ray

Chest radiography is the examination of first choice. MS can present in several different ways, the most common of which is a homogeneous left posterobasal opacity, which may or may not be associated with cystic plaques within the opacity. This location is suggestive of the diagnosis [6,5,11]. However, the type of radiological abnormality is not an element of orientation, as a cystic or hydro-

preload [63]. Despite its effectiveness in a case of pulmonary sequestration, he acknowledged the absence of pharmacological data in the fretus, and the possible passage into maternal blood. He thought, however, that this could reduce the frequency of thoracocentesis.

All fretus surgery carries risks of premature rupture of membranes, premature delivery, chorioamniotitis and maternal-fretal infection. However, any intervention on the fretus should only be considered if there is an immediate vital risk to the fretus.

b- Open fretal surgery

If the systemic vessel has never been identified, it may not be accessible for treatment. In the absence of hydrothorax, only open surgical removal of the vessel can be envisaged [64]. Neonatal survival of around 50% can be expected [65]. However, this therapeutic option involves high risks not only for the current pregnancy, but also for the mother and any subsequent pregnancy.

In our series, none of the patients had prenatal treatment.

3 Post-natal treatment

a- Surgical treatment

It is the cornerstone of treatment and is based on a lobectomy or segmentectomy for SIL, and an elective exeresis (sequestrectomy) for SEL [23].

The age at which surgery should be performed is a subject of controversy. Some authors recommend surgery at an early age, to avoid compression of the growing pulmonary alveoli by the malformation [66,67,68].

i. Preparing the patient

This is a major operation involving contact with the large vessels in the thorax, with a potential risk of sudden bleeding. A pre-operative blood test should include blood grouping, a blood count and a haemostasis test. Similarly, a supply of iso-rhesus blood, if possible phenotyped outside the emergency department, is essential.

If there is any suspicion of associated cardiovascular malformation, a cardiac ultrasound scan should be ordered to guide treatment.

ii. Approach

S **<u>Thoracotomy</u>**

This is usually a posterolateral thoracotomy. The fifth intercostal space is chosen because of the frequency of localisations in the lower lobe. The main advantage of this approach is vascular control. Control of the systemic artery is the main danger in sequestration surgery. This is sometimes a large-calibre artery that can be more than half the diameter of the aorta, with an elastic component that does not have the spasm capacity of the more peripheral systemic arteries. The other advantage is exploration of the pleural cavity, with

the possibility of palpating the lung parenchyma. The disadvantages are functional, with more post-operative pain than with a minimally invasive approach, and the risk of musculoskeletal deformities due to asymmetry of the thoracic cage, scoliosis and costal synostosis [71]. The aesthetic consequences for the skin are not negligible.
Before the thoracotomy, the patient should be positioned in a lateral decubitus position, leaning slightly forward, with the homolateral upper limb raised, allowing the scapula to be spread and the muscles to relax. A sub-costal block is placed to widen the inter-costal spaces. The surgeon is positioned on the patient's back, while the assistant is on the front of the thorax [72].

S **Thoracoscopy**

Although thoracoscopy was first proposed in children in the mid-1970s by B. Rodgers as an aid to diagnosis and lung biopsies, it is only in the last two decades that we have seen its development in the therapeutic field [73,74]. This approach to MS is increasingly being reported [73,75]. In 1994, Watine et al. reported the first case to be operated on thoracoscopically. The patient is always positioned in lateral decubitus on the opposite side to the lesion, with a block placed beforehand, which allows a good view of the hilum anteriorly and posteriorly.
The operator, the optic, the area to be operated on and the monitor must all be placed on the same line, with the optic implantation site as the axis of rotation [74].
The position of the optic is generally between the tip of the scapula and the anterior axillary line at the 4eme or 5eme intercostal space, or the intersection between the anterior axillary line and the 5eme or 6 ^{eme}intercostal space. A pneumothorax will be created by insufflation of CO2, causing the lungs to collapse and creating a working space.
There are usually 2 to 5 operating trocars, positioned in triangulation and behind the anterior axillary line.
Despite the fact that it is impossible to palpate the lung parenchyma, thoracoscopy offers excellent visibility of the pleural cavity, particularly at the level of the costodiaphragmatic sinus, a possible site of passage for the systemic artery, the identification of which is the main difficulty. This visibility, and therefore the comfort of the surgical procedure, is however dependent on good homolateral pulmonary exclusion, especially for SIL. There is no greater morbidity or mortality than with thoracotomy [76]. In addition to the aesthetic advantages, there is less post-operative pain and hospital stay, and in the longer term fewer musculoskeletal consequences [77, 78].
Conversion to thoracotomy remains an option, of course, particularly in the

event of vascular or anaesthetic problems, or operative difficulties (adhesions, major intestinal dilatation, etc.).
In a Chinese study, Liu reported 18 cases of MS treated thoracoscopically (2 SEL, 16 SIL), of which only one case of SEL was converted to thoracotomy because of a lesion of the systemic artery with the occurrence of a large hemothorax [78].
In our series, thoracoscopy was chosen in 8 patients (50%), but this approach enabled MS to be treated in 31.25% of cases (5 patients). The reasons for conversion were uncontrollable bleeding in one case and dissection difficulties in the remaining 2 cases.

iii. Operating time proper

There are two stages in the procedure, which are progressively divided into exploration and treatment.
The first and most important stage in lung sequestration surgery is control of the systemic vessel.

***S* The** main aim of **surgical exploration** is to visualise and identify the feeding artery. The artery must be controlled very carefully, given the fragility of its embryonic wall and its elasticity. This means that optimal control is required to avoid retraction into the mediastinum or through the aortic orifice of the diaphragm, making control difficult or even impossible. Some cases of fatal intraoperative haemorrhage have been described when the diagnosis is unknown, which always requires careful palpation and dissection of the triangular ligament [2]. Exploration of the entire pleural cavity is of course indicated, as well as the mediastinum. It may be associated with another MBP (MAKP, bronchogenic cyst), or a diaphragmatic hernia, which should be treated at the same time, or biopsied depending on the per-operative findings.

***S* Sequestrectomy**

MS is best treated by elective exeresis, as this malformation is well separated from the normal lung by its own pleural envelope. No parenchymal section is required. The SEL has an arterio-venous pedicle, or even a broncho-arterio-venous pedicle if it communicates with the digestive tract. The pedicle must therefore be dissected, and the ligation-section of each element performed separately. These principles apply to intra-thoracic, intra-diaphragmatic and sub-diaphragmatic SEL [39].
In our series, sequestrectomy was performed in 11 cases of SEL.

***S* Lobectomy**

This is the treatment of choice for SIL. Once control of the systemic artery has been achieved by ligation-section, resection depends on the location, and is more or less typical and systematised [79].

Lobectomy must comply with the general rules for pulmonary surgery. This involves the following stages:

- Dissection of the pedicle and the accessible scissure
- Ligation of arteries after they have been identified
- Ligation of superficial veins
- Dissection of the bronchus is an important step which should only be carried out once the topography has been correctly identified to avoid any errors [80].

After exercise, two imperatives must be respected [80,81]:

- Aerostasis and hemostasis of the pleural slice is necessary.

The airtightness of the bronchial suture is checked by immersing the bronchial stump in physiological serum.

- One or two pleural drains are inserted, while checking that they are working properly.

***S* Segmentectomy**

It is rarely indicated [82].

In our series, no patient underwent segmentectomy.

***S* Right or left pneumonectomy**

They are exceptionally indicated, but are necessary in cases of sequestration of the entire lung [83].

b- Endovascular treatment

Some authors suggest treating only the systemic vascular anomaly without resecting the MS, i.e. obliterating the systemic artery as the sole treatment for sequestration [84].

i. Principles

By occluding the systemic artery, some authors hope that the sequestration will regress or even disappear. This procedure is based on the observation of cases of pulmonary sequestration which have spontaneously involuted, either in the antenatal period [20] and/or postnatally [85]. This spontaneous involution and disappearance is attributed to infarction of the MBP [85]. Of course, this therapeutic option has the advantage of being less invasive than thoracotomy, the main argument put forward by its advocates.

ii. Methods and approaches

Although thoracoscopic ligation was reported by Watine in 1994, embolisation is currently being developed in some centres. The occlusive agents used are mainly coils [86-87]. The problem arises more in terms of the arterial access route, especially in the very young. In addition to the common femoral route, some authors suggest catheterisation of the umbilical artery in newborns [88].

iii. Indications

Embolisation of the systemic artery is a solution to consider in the event of cardiac failure with hemodynamic instability, or in the event of hemoptysis [86]. Some authors have reported cases of embolisation prior to surgical resection, in order to reduce the risk of haemorrhage [86]. Embolisation as a curative treatment for MS is advocated by some authors in view of the possibility of spontaneous regression [85]. Embolisation could be justified in asymptomatic children with MS and probably of reasonable size. Its less invasive aspect is emphasised, but it is not without complications. This treatment needs to be evaluated in terms of indications, age at which it should be performed, complications and radiological follow-up methods, in order to limit radiation exposure in these children.

iv. Complications

The local complications of catheterisation of the common femoral artery are hematoma at the puncture site, arteriovenous fistula, and above all thrombosis, the immediate consequence of which is acute ischaemia of the limb [88].

Thrombo-embolic complications may occur at a distance from the puncture site, and therefore also following catheterisation of the umbilical artery. Adelman reported a case of long-lasting hypertension following such a procedure, with thrombosis of the renal artery and secondary renal atrophy [89].

Following the procedure, transient arterial hypertension may occur, probably of thrombo-embolic origin, as well as pain, hyperthermia, or reactive pleurisy. The coils may also migrate, repermeabilising the systemic artery [89].

Therapeutic management of sequestration by embolisation requires closer and more prolonged radiological follow-up than surgical treatment. This follow-up is imperative in the case of a sequestration left in place, especially as embolisation is not 100% effective, either because the artery is repermeabilised or because there is an additional non-embolised artery [86].

In the literature, the failure rate is estimated at between 15 and 80% [18].

In our series, no child benefited from endovascular treatment.

4. Therapeutic indications

a- Indications for in utero treatment

Antenatal suspicion of MS requires regular monitoring with more frequent ultrasound scans to monitor the progress of the lesion.

If the lesion stabilises or regresses, regular monitoring of the pregnancy is sufficient, and delivery should be scheduled in a 3eme level maternity hospital to ensure better care for the newborn [27].

Frequent intervention could be considered in the event of complications and in the absence of other associated malformations or chromosomal aberrations [90]. The aim is to preserve freight life and avoid the development of irreversible pulmonary hypoplasia and pulmonary arterial hypertension [91]. The decision must be a multidisciplinary one involving the paediatric surgeon, obstetrician and anaesthetist. An interview with the parents and a discussion of the benefits and risks are necessary.

In the case of polyhydramnios with major mediastinal deviation, repeated amniocentesis, pleural fretal drainage and thoracoamniotic shunting under video-endoscopic or ultrasound control may be proposed [27, 46,59,91].

Fretal lobectomy is an alternative if there is no improvement [64].

From 32 weeks' amenorrhoea, premature delivery is required for post-natal exeresis [65,92].

Therapeutic complications are dominated by rupture of membranes, premature delivery, chorio-amniotitis, side effects of tocolytics and the need for cesarean delivery in subsequent pregnancies.

b- Post-natal treatment

Who to operate

> Symptomatic forms

In symptomatic patients, there is unanimous agreement on the indication for therapy [18].

> Asymptomatic forms

While the indication for treatment of symptomatic MS is clear, the treatment of asymptomatic MS remains a subject of controversy [18]. Some believe that the risk of surgery is greater than the risk of complications [18,44].

Other authors advocate early treatment for a number of reasons. Firstly, there is the risk of complications, especially lung infections, making removal of the malformation more difficult and the post-operative course less straightforward. In addition, early removal of the malformation should allow optimal growth of the healthy lung, which is still compressed by the lesion [93]. However, there was a lack of clear evidence of benefit between preventive surgery and the conservative approach in asymptomatic patients.

Prospective multicentre studies, at best randomised, with a long follow-up period, can help optimise the management of asymptomatic forms.

When to operate?

Symptomatic forms pose no problem, as it is accepted that there is no age limit.

For asymptomatic forms, there is no conventional age for surgery. However, the larger the malformation, the earlier the operation should be.

On the other hand, if there is any etiological doubt, surgery is essential, as other malformations (MAKP) are at risk of cancer.

In our series, asymptomatic patients were operated on as soon as the diagnosis was strongly suspected on imaging.

What is the approach?

The feasibility of thoracoscopy depends on the patient's general condition and the surgeon's experience.

This approach can aggravate pre-existing respiratory insufficiency and vascular collapse by increasing intra-thoracic pressure.

On the other hand, the small working space in neonates and small infants makes it difficult to control the vascular ligation and conversion may be necessary [94].

In our series, 5 patients underwent successful thoracoscopic surgery, while 3 patients required conversion to thoracotomy.

What is the role of post-operative pleural drainage?

While SIL involves a lobectomy with scissural dissection requiring drainage, SEL involves only a simple sequestrectomy and may not require drainage. In fact, it is a matter of team choice. For some patients, drainage is systematic and its purpose is to drain the air and fluid, which makes it possible to control or detect any complications, especially bleeding complications, and often a single chest tube. On the other hand, drainage is an entry point for nosocomial infections and increases the post-operative stay [95].

In our series, all patients underwent postoperative chest drainage.

VII. ANATOMOPATHOLOGICAL STUDY

1. **Macroscopic appearance**

> SIL

The SIL appears macroscopically as a pinkish or yellowish mass with a clear boundary with the normally aerated neighbouring segment. The parenchyma is often atelectatic or dystrophic [96].

> SEL

SEL appears macroscopically as an accessory lung mass, independent of the rest of the lung parenchyma. Its appearance is hepatized, violaceous and non-aerosic [96].

2. **Microscopic aspect**

Microscopically, the sequestrum consists of several cavities with either a bronchial structure or a collagenous wall covered with cylindrical or flattened epithelium. Areas of atelectasis or alveolar dysplasia may be present [2,23].

3. **Histology of the systemic artery**

The artery vascularising a pulmonary sequestration is a systemic artery and has a thicker wall than a pulmonary artery.

[3,23]. It is a resistant, elastic artery which can retract if transected.

In our series, surgical exploration and anatomopathological examination corrected the diagnosis made on imaging in 8 patients (8/16), thus confirming the diagnosis of MS.

VII. DIAGNOSTIC PROBLEMS

Errors in diagnosis arise from antenatal life, when variable and non-specific images are seen on antenatal ultrasound. Post-natally, the clinical and radiological pictures are variable and sometimes misleading. The problem arises when a cystic formation is localized to a lobe [32].

1. Adenomatous cystic pulmonary malformation

MAKP are the most common congenital lung malformations. They are characterised by adenomatoid proliferation of the bronchiolar structures and the formation of single or multiple cysts. This is the main differential diagnosis for MS. The 2 malformations are sometimes associated within the same lesion, thus forming hybrid MS [42,43,44].

2. Bronchogenic cyst

It may or may not communicate with the tracheobronchial tree. It is characterised by a predilection for the lower lobes. The radiological appearance is that of a rounded homogeneous opacity with a watery tone and regular contours, often unique. A hydroaerobic level may be seen if there is communication with the tracheobronchial tree [97,98].

3. Arteriovenous malformation

It is discussed when an aberrant systemic artery is visualised [11]. It is a differential diagnosis, especially with Pryce's type I MS.

4. Other

Other diagnoses may be discussed, such as a lung tumour, mediastinal teratoma or digestive duplication (particularly cystic resophagus) [97,98,99,100].

The clinical and radiological polymorphism of pulmonary sequestration leads to diagnostic and therapeutic difficulties. This illustrates the diagnostic difficulties that clinicians and even radiologists can face. Management is based on multidisciplinary collaboration between paediatricians, paediatric surgeons, radiologists and pathologists. The diagnosis of certainty is made by surgical and anatomopathological exploration.

VIII. EVOLUTION

The outcome of surgical treatment is generally favourable. Rarely, however, complications may arise.

1. Simple operating sequences

They are observed in the majority of cases, with good tolerance of extubation and disappearance of respiratory signs and radiological abnormalities [28].

2. Intraoperative complications

Intra-operatively, the complications may be vascular, with injury to the systemic artery during dissection, particularly in a fibro-inflammatory environment, possibly associated with vascular retraction into the posterior mediastinum or sub-diaphragm. This complication is the most feared, especially as this artery is by definition elastic, and therefore lacks the capacity for vasospasm. The wound may involve the aorta, particularly as the artery may be short [101]. In any event, dissection of the artery must be cautious and sufficient to allow double ligation and vascular sectioning, sparing an upstream stump, rather than pushing towards the parenchymal side [78].

The other complications are those of any lung resection, particularly in the case of larger parenchymal resections such as lobectomies, with difficulties that may arise during control of the pulmonary artery or pulmonary vein concerned.

In our series, we reported a case of major intraoperative bleeding requiring conversion to thoracotomy.

3. Post-operative complications

Immediate post-operative morbidity can be as high as 28% [102,103]. The main complications to be feared are hemothorax secondary to haemorrhage at the level of the arterial stump, and persistent air leaks which may require prolonged pleural drainage. Pleural empyema may also occur in the postoperative period, particularly after superinfectious sequestration [102,104]. These complications may occur whatever the approach.

4. Long-term results

Long-term post-operative outcome is favourable in the majority of cases, especially in the absence of associated malformations, mainly cardiovascular, which may be life-threatening [102].

> Clinical aspects

Most operated patients are asymptomatic post-operatively. This is explained by the existence of an adaptation mechanism a few months to a few years after lobectomy. In rare cases, a cough and/or wheezing may be observed and regress after a few months or years [32,105,106].

In our series, all our patients were asymptomatic with an average follow-up of 9 years.

> Radiology

The chest X-ray is often normal, with parenchymal expansion becoming more complete the earlier the surgery [32].

> Functional and spirometric aspects

Respiratory function tests may show either a restrictive syndrome proportional to the lung volume resected, or an amputation of volumes below the resected volume, confirming the theory of compensatory alveolar growth, or finally an increase in the ratio of residual volume to total lung capacity, an indicator of distension [107].

> **Orthopaedic braces**

They are dominated by dystrophies of the thoracic wall and scoliosis, observed after extensive lung resection. Some teams propose the use of intrathoracic expanders, the volume of which can be modified according to growth. The aim of these expanders is essentially to limit secondary scoliosis [108].

> **Aesthetic seams**

They are characterised by thoracic asymmetry, or an anomaly in the growth or position of the mammary gland, which must be screened, as treatment with a prosthesis may be proposed after the end of puberty.

The thoracotomy scar may be unsightly, and thoracoscopy is the best means of prevention [108].

In our series, no orhtopedic sequelae were observed. The appearance of the scar was satisfactory. Functional respiratory exploration was not performed.

5. Monitoring

> **In non-operated forms**, the patient is monitored clinically and radiologically. The aim is to detect complications and recommend surgery in good time.

> The surveillance methods **used** are the same.

The aim is to look for post-operative complications and treat them early, before any sequelae appear. Our patients were monitored closely at first, every 3 to 6 months, then annually. Subsequently, respiratory function tests were performed to assess functional results.

As we have already seen, pulmonary sequestration remains a complex pathology. In fact, its pre-operative and even per-operative diagnosis is sometimes difficult. Diagnosis of this bronchopulmonary malformation and identification of the vascular pedicle, especially the aberrant systemic artery, remains a real challenge. As a result, we can see that centralising this pathology in a single specialised centre would be appropriate, in order to better identify and control the diagnosis of pulmonary sequestration, thus enabling ideal management.

Conclusion

I. Introduction

Pulmonary sequestration (PS) is a rare bronchopulmonary malformation, defined as a non-functioning lung territory that has lost its normal bronchial and

vascular connections.
Advances in imaging and surgery, particularly thoracoscopy, have prompted this original study, which aims to contribute to the anatomical-clinical-radiological study of this malformative pathology using data reported by the various professionals involved, namely paediatricians, paediatric radiologists, paediatric surgeons and anatomopathologists.
From a retrospective study of 16 cases of MS diagnosed and treated in the department of pediatric surgery in Monastir over a period of 29 years from 1990 to 2019, we tried to :

- to clarify the etiopathogenic aspects of pulmonary sequestration,
- study the epidemiological and clinical features,
- explain the elements of radiological diagnosis,

-compare the diagnoses made on imaging with the results of the pathological examination,

- discuss the different approaches to lung sequestration surgery in children,
- and discuss the diagnostic problems that may arise with other congenital or acquired conditions.

II. Materials and methods:

This is a retrospective descriptive study of 16 observations of pulmonary sequestration in the paediatric surgery department of the Fattouma Bourguiba Hospital in Monastir. Information was collected from medical records, radiological and operative reports. The positive diagnosis was based on the anatomopathological study.

III. Results

Our series included 7 boys and 9 girls. The mean age was 30 months. MS was detected before birth in 8 of 16 cases (50%), at a median term of 21 weeks' amenorrhoea, and was strongly suggested by visualisation of an aberrant systemic artery in 2 of 8 cases (25%).
Three newborns and 2 infants were diagnosed antenatally with MBP and were symptomatic. These were severe neonatal respiratory distress requiring mechanical ventilation in 2 cases (cases 2, 4), moderate in one case (case 12), acute bronchiolitis in one case (case 7) and febrile bronchopneumopathy in the remaining case (case 16).
In these patients, surgery was scheduled. In addition, 3 patients aged 1, 3 and 18 months respectively (cases 1, 3, 15), in whom antenatal imaging had suspected MBP, were asymptomatic. Given the absence of functional signs and the absence of signs of ultrasound severity during antenatal imaging (pleural effusion, mediastinal deviation), the decision was made to monitor them clinically and radiologically without immediate recourse to surgery, until a

precise diagnosis was made.

In the absence of antenatal diagnosis, 2 patients presented with acute bronchiolitis, whereas 3 presented with febrile pneumonitis.

In the 3 remaining cases (cases 9, 10, 13), pulmonary sequestration was the result of incidental discovery of a herniated diaphragmatic dome during surgery.

All our patients had a chest X-ray. This examination was performed from birth in the case of antenatal diagnosis. For the other patients, the chest X-ray was performed on the occasion of a respiratory warning sign. It showed parenchymal opacity in 4 patients (4/16) (25%), of left postero-basal origin in 1 case/4 and occupying the right pulmonary hemichampus in 3 cases/4. In addition, it showed left para-cardiac opacity in 2 cases/16 (12.5%), posterior, retro-cardiac opacity in one case/16, left apical clearing in one case and pulmonary parenchymal condensation in 3 cases/16 (18.75%). In 3 patients (3/16) (18.75%), it showed intrathoracic digestive clartes.

In addition, in 2 patients (2/16), the chest X-ray showed a large pleural effusion. After pleural drainage, the diagnosis of bronchopulmonary malformation was suspected, in the absence of clinical improvement.

Thoracic CT angiography suggested the diagnosis of pulmonary sequestration in 7 patients (7/16) (43.75%), showing pulmonary parenchymal condensation fed by systemic arterial branches in 4 cases/16 (25%) and a mediastinal tissue mass fed by an artery from the descending aorta and drained by a systemic vein in 3 cases/16 (18.75%). Among these patients, MAKP was associated with MS in 2 cases.

The other diagnoses given were isolated MAKP in 2 cases (12.50%), bronchogenic cyst or pleuropericardial cyst or resophageal duplication in one case, MAKP associated with bronchogenic cyst in one case. Only one patient was operated on with a diagnosis of hydatid cyst of the lung. In addition, herniation of the left diaphragmatic dome without any other associated malformation was diagnosed in 3 patients (18.75%). Finally, a pleural effusion was found in only one case, without any underlying cause or associated malformation.

Thoracic MRI angiography was carried out in a single patient, and showed a left posterobasal lung parenchymal condensation, with a T1 iso-signal and moderate T2 hyper-signal, fed by systemic vessels.

On the imaging data, the malformation involved the left side in 12 cases/16 (75%) and the right side in 4 cases/16 (25%).

All children underwent surgery. The open approach was performed in 8 children (8/16) (50%) by a posterolateral thoracotomy centred on the 5eme intercostal space.

Thoracoscopy was attempted in 8 patients (8/16) (50%). This approach enabled MS to be treated in 31.25% of cases (5 cases/16).
The reasons for conversion were the occurrence of uncontrollable bleeding in one case and dissection difficulties in the remaining 2 cases. The procedure of choice was sequestrectomy in SEL (11 cases/16) and lobectomy in SIL and hybrid forms (5 cases/16).
All pieces of surgery were sent for histological study.
Anatomopathological examination confirmed the diagnosis of pulmonary sequestration. Sequestration was intra-lobar in 4 of 16 cases (25%) and extra-lobar in 12 of 16 cases (75%). All patients had a favourable post-operative outcome. There was no mortality. The mean follow-up was 9 years.

Discussion:

Pulmonary sequestration is a bronchopulmonary malformation secondary to an anomaly occurring during pulmonary organogenesis. It accounts for 0.15 to 6.14% of pulmonary malformations. MS was first described by Rokitanski in 1861, but it was Pryce who, in 1946, gave a precise definition, introduced the term sequestration and proposed a classification into intra- and extra-lobar. In 75% of cases, SPs lie between the diaphragm and the lower lobe (80% on the left).
There are two types of pulmonary sequestration:

- Extra-lobar sequestration (25%): the SEL is surrounded by its own visceral vein without communicating with the tracheobronchial tree. It is often associated with other malformations, the most common of which are diaphragmatic hernias, cystic adenomatoid malformations and bronchogenic cysts.
- Intra-lobar sequestration: the non-functional tissue is included in the lung parenchyma and enveloped by the normal pleural envelope.

The development of pulmonary sequestration occurs early in gestational life between 5eme and 6eme weeks gestation. Pryce's theory is the most widely adopted at present. It is based on a vascular theory relating to aberrant, persistent systemic vascularisation, which is responsible for the pulmonary malformation.
The diagnosis of pulmonary sequestration is a difficult one. The clinical signs are not specific and the anomaly remains latent for a long time. It is suggested on the basis of anamnestic and clinical elements combined with imaging data. It is essential that the abnormal arterial vascularisation (main and collateral arteries) and even the venous drainage of the sequestrated zone are identified to confirm the diagnosis and guide the therapeutic management, which is usually surgical. A frontal thoracic X-ray may be helpful in making the diagnosis in the presence of posterobasal opacity, particularly on the left. Contrast-enhanced CT

is an excellent examination for the diagnosis and pre-operative assessment of pulmonary sequestration. It recognises the nature of the mass and shows the systemic artery. In our series, CT angiography showed pulmonary parenchymal condensation fed by systemic arterial branches in 4 cases (25%). In 3 patients (18.75%), it showed a mediastinal tissue mass fed by an artery from the descending aorta and drained by a systemic vein.
Aortography is no longer used for diagnostic purposes, and is now reserved for embolisation techniques. Treatment of pulmonary sequestration is essentially surgical. Control of the systemic feeder artery is tricky, given the fragility of its embryonic wall and its elasticity, with the risk of retraction into the mediastinum or through the diaphragm. Surgery often consists of lobectomy in SIL and sequestrectomy in SEL. Thoracoscopy appears to be technically more feasible for extra-lobar sequestration. In our series, we opted for thoracoscopy in 8 patients, with conversion in 3 cases. The reasons for conversion were uncontrollable bleeding in one case and dissection difficulties in the remaining 2 cases. Endo-vascular techniques are currently proposed for the treatment of pulmonary sequestration, mainly in patients in poor general condition or with heart failure. This technique may not be sufficient, in which case it must be supplemented by a surgical procedure.
While surgical indication cannot be discussed in symptomatic patients, given the risk of sudden, unpredictable and dramatic decompensation, the increase in antenatal diagnosis in asymptomatic forms means that the conservative approach is debatable, at the cost of close, vigilant clinical and radiological monitoring. This approach remains controversial, with different attitudes depending on the author.
Fetal fret therapy is a recent modality under development, ranging from amniocentesis to fetal lobectomy. It is indicated in cases of polyhydramnios with major mediastinal deviation, but is not without risk.
If treated early, MS has a good prognosis. Progression after surgical treatment is generally favourable. Finally, by teaching young surgeons how to use thoracoscopy, these patients can be operated on in complete safety. This is made possible by advances in anaesthesia and paediatric resuscitation.
Conclusion: Pulmonary sequestration can take on different radio-clinical forms, sometimes leading to confusion. Although imaging has made constant progress, there are still diagnostic difficulties. Confirmation remains anatomopathological by analysing the surgical specimen.
In short, the creation of a centre specialising in surgery for bronchopulmonary malformations seems obvious, with a common objective: to organise better care for children. This project is based on

coordinating the various players involved: obstetricians, neonatologists, paediatricians, radiologists, paediatric surgeons and pathologists.

APPENDIX

APPENDIX DATA COLLECTION FORM

- Population characteristics
- Full name
- Date of birth
- Gender
- Data from the interview
- Family history of bronchopulmonary malformation.s
- Pregnancy course and antenatal ultrasound data
- antenatal diagnosis of pulmonary anomaly)
- Perinatal incidents
- Time between onset of signs and positive diagnosis.
- Circumstances of discovery
- Antenatal diagnosis
- Respiratory distress
- Dyspnea
- Cough
- Broncho-pneumonia
- Per-operative
- Data from the clinical examination
- Polypnee
- Signs of struggle
- Reductions in vesicular murmurs
- Rales on auscultation
- Fever
- Associated deformities
- Data from additional tests
- Chest X-ray, front and side view
- Thoracic Doppler ultrasound
- Thoracic angiography and modelling
- Surgical treatment
- Approach
- Operational findings

- Gestures
- Incidents
- Drainage
- Anatomopathological findings
- Post-operative complications
- Development and results
- Mortality

References

1- Aloui-kasbi N, Bellagha I, Hammou A. Pulmonary sequestration: particular clinical and radiological features. Arch Pediatr 2004;11:394-6.

2- Kabiri H, Smahi M, Achir A, Herrak L, Alaziz S, Elmeslout A et al. Pulmonary sequestration. A propos de 5 cas. Med Maghr 2000;83: 7-12.

3- Pryce DM. Lower accessory pulmonary artery with intralobar sequestration of lung; a report of seven cases. J Pathol Bacteriol 1946;58:457-67.

4- Clements BS, Warner JO. Pulmonary sequestration and related congenital bronchopulmonary-vascular malformations: nomenclature and classification based on anatomical and embryological considerations. Thorax 1987;42:401-8.

5- Zhang SX, Wang HD, Yang K, Cheng W, Wu W. Retrospective review of the diagnosis and treatment of pulmonary sequestration in 28 patients: surgery or endovascular techniques? J Thorac Dis 2017;9:5153-60.

6- Qian X, Sun Y, Liu D, Wu X, Wang Z, Tang Y. Pulmonary sequestration: a case report and literature review. Int J Clin Exp Med 2015;8:21822-5.

7- Bousetta K, Aloui-Kasbi N, Fitouri Z, Sammoud A, Becher SB, Hammou A et al. Congenital lung malformations: contribution of imaging. J Pediatr Pueric 2004;17:370-9.

8- Salles M, Deschildre A, Bonnel C, Dubos JP, Bonnevalle M, Devismes L et al. Diagnosis and treatment of congenital bronchopulmonary malformations: analysis of 32 observations. Arch Pediatr 2005;12:1703-8.

9- Wei Y, Li F. Pulmonary sequestration: a retrospective analysis of 2625 cases in China. Eur J Cardiothorac Surg 2011;40:e39-42.

10- Berteloot L, Bobbio A, Millischer-Bellaiche AE, Lambot K, Breton S, Brunelle F. Congenital lung malformations, the radiologist's point of view. Revue des Maladies Respiratoires 2012;29:820-35.

11- Walker CM, Wu CC, Gilman MD, Godwin JD, Shepard JA, et al. The imaging spectrum of bronchopulmonary sequestration. Curr Probl Diagn Radiol 2014;43:100-14.

12- Kolls JK, Kiernan MP, Ascuitto RJ, Ross-Ascuitto NT, Fox LS. Intralobar pulmonary sequestration presenting as congestive heart failure in a neonate. Chest 1992;102:974-6.

13- Frazier AA, Rosado de Christenson ML, Stocker JT, Templeton PA. Intralobar sequestration: radiologic-pathologic correlation. Radiographics 1997;17:725-45.

14- Tashtoush B, Memarpour R, Gonzalez J, Gleason JB, Hadeh A. Pulmonary sequestration: a 29 patient case series and review. J Clin Diagn Res 2015;9:05-8.

15- Savic B, Birtel FJ, Tholen W, Funke HD, Knoche R. Lung sequestration: report of seven cases and review of 540 published cases. Thorax. 1979;34:96-

101.
16- Corbett HJ, Humphrey GME. Pulmonary sequestration. Paediatr Respir Rev 2004;5:59-68.
17- Al-Salem AH. An Illustrated Guide to Pediatric Surgery. Pulmonary Sequestration Chapter 53 2014;393-399.
18- Khen-Dunlop N, Farmakis K, Berteloot L, Gobbo F, Stirnemann J, De Blic J et al. Bronchopulmonary sequestrations in a paediatric centre: ongoing practices and debated management. Eur J Cardiothorac Surg 2018;54:246-51.
19- Ou J, Lei X, Fu Z, Huang Y, Liu E, Luo Z, et al. Pulmonary sequestration in children: a clinical analysis of 48 cases. Int J Clin Exp Med 2014;7:1355-65.
20- Gezer S, Ta stepe I, Sirmali M, Findik G, Turut H, Kaya **S** et al. Pulmonary sequestration: a single-institutional series composed of 27 cases. J Thorac Cardiovasc Surg 2007;133:955-9.
21- Van Raemdonck D, De Boeck K, Devlieger H, Demedts M, Moerman P, Coosemans W et al. Pulmonary sequestration: a comparison between pediatric and adult patients. Eur J Cardiothorac Surg 2001;19:388-395.
22- Halkic N, Cuenoud PF, Corthesy ME, Ksontini R, Boumghar M. Pulmonary sequestration: a review of 26 cases. Eur J Cardiothorac Surg 1998;14:127-33.
23- Kabiri H, Atoini F, Zidane A, Jidal M, Arsalane A, Rguibi M et al. Sequestration of the posterobasal segment of the right lower lung lobe. Annales de Chirurgie 2006;131: 547-549.
24- Sane SM, Girdany BR. Cysts and neoplasms in the infant lung. Semin. Roentgenol 1972;7:25-32.
25- Ben Abdallah R, Bouthour H, Hellal Y, Ben Malek R, Gharbi Y, Kaabar N. Les Malformations Broncho-Pulmonaires: Aspects
radiological and therapeutic diagnostics. La tunisie medicale 2013;91:66-9.
26- Hourrier S, Salomon L.J, Bault J.P, Dumez Y, Ville Y. Congenital lung malformations: antenatal diagnosis and management . Rev Mal Respir 2011;28:1017-24.
27- Lecomte B, Hadden H, Coste K, Gallot D, Laurichesse H, Lemery D et al. Hyperechoic congenital lung lesions in a non-selected population: from prenatal detection till perinatal management. Prenat Diagn 2009; 29:1222-30.
28- Truitt AK, Carr SR, Cassese J, Kurkchubasche AG, Tracy TF Jr, Luks FI. Perinatal management of congenital cystic lung lesions in the age of minimally invasive surgery. J Pediatr Surg 2006;41:893-6.
29- Corbett HJ, Humphrey GM. Pulmonary sequestration. Paediatr Respir Rev 2004;5:59-68.
30- Nagar R, Butter A, Brahm G, Price A. Pulmonary sequestration causing severe cardiac failure requiring lobectomy in an extreme preterm infant. J

Pediatr Surg Case Rep 2015;3:415-8.
31- Divjak N, Vasseur Maurer S, Giannoni E, Vial Y, de Buys Roessingh A, Wildhaber BE. Bronchopulmonary Sequestration with Morbid Neonatal Pleural Effusion despite Successful Antenatal Treatment. Front Pediatr 2017;5:259.
32- Khemiri M, Khaldi F, Hamzaoui A, Chaouachi B, Hamzaoui M, Ben Becher S et al. Cystic pulmonary malformations: clinical and radiological polymorphism. A propos de 30 observations. Rev Pneumol Clin 2009;65:333-40.
33- Durand Ch, Garel C, Nugues F, Baudain P. L'echographie dans la pathologie thoracique de l'enfant. Journal de radiologie 2001;82: 729-737.
34- Mama N, Dhifallah M, Ben Aicha S, Kadri K, Arifa N, Hasni I et al. CT imaging of excised lung lesions. Feuill Radiol 2014;54:69-83.
35- Lee EY, Dillon JE, Callahan MJ, Voss SD. 3D multidetector CT angiographic evaluation of extralobar pulmonary sequestration with anomalous venous drainage into the left internal mammary vein in a paediatric patient. Br J Radiol 2006;79:e99-102.
36- Berrocal T, Madrid C, Novo S, Gutierrez J, Arjonilla A, GomezLeon N. Congenital anomalies of the tracheobronchial tree, lung, and mediastinum: embryology, radiology, and pathology. Radiographics 2004;24:e17.
37- Lee CK, Lee CH, Baliski C, Zetler P. Retroperitoneal extralobar pulmonary sequestration mimicking a pheochromocytoma. Histopathology 2008;52:525-7.
38- Lin CH, Chuang CY, Hsia JY, Lee MC, Shai SE, Yang SS, et al. Pulmonary sequestration-differences in diagnosis and treatment in a single institution. J Chin Med Assoc 2013;76:385-9.
39- Sancak T, Cangir AK, Atasoy C, Ozdemir N. The role of contrast enhanced three-dimensional MR angiography in pulmonary sequestration. Interact Cardiovasc Thorac Surg 2003;2:480-2.
40- Sauvanet A, Regnard JF, Calanducci F, Rojas-Miranda A, Dartevelle P, Levasseur P. Pulmonary sequestration. Surgical aspects based on 61 cases. Rev Pneumol Clin 1991;47:126-132.
41- Yue SW, Guo H, Zhang YG, Gao JB, Ma XX, Ding PX. The clinical value of computer tomographic angiography for the diagnosis and therapeutic planning of patients with pulmonary sequestration. Eur J Cardiothorac Surg 2013;43:946-51.
42- Conran RM, Stocker JT. Extralobar sequestration with frequently associated congenital cystic adenomatoid malformation, type 2: report of 50 cases. Pediatr Dev Pathol 1999;2:454-63.
43- Cebeci B, Erener-Ercan T, Babayigit A, Agirgol E, Buyukkale G, Qetinkaya.M. Co-Existence of Congenital Cystic Adenomatoid Malformation

and Pulmonary Sequestration in a Newborn with Spontaneous Pneumothorax: A Case Report and Review of the Literature. Med Bull Haseki 2019;57:211-214.

44- Orpen N, Goodman R, Bowker C, Lakhoo K. Intralobar pulmonary sequestration with congenital cystic adematous malformation and rhabdomyomatous dysplasia. Pediatr Surg Int. 2003;19(8):610-1.

45- Nunes C, Pereira I, Araujo C, Santo SF, Carvalho RM, Melo A et al. Fetal bronchopulmonary malformations. J Matern Fetal Neonatal Med 2015;28:1996-2000.

46- Mallmann MR, Geipel A, Bludau M, Matil K, Gottschalk I, Hoopmann M et al. Bronchopulmonary sequestration with massive pleural effusion: pleuroamniotic shunting vs intrafetal vascular laser ablation. Ultrasound Obstet Gynecol 2014; 44:441.

47- Delacourt C, Remy-Jardin M, Revillon Y, Piegay F. Treatment of bronchopulmonary malformations in children. Rev Mal Respir Actual 2011;3:158-61.

48- Cavoretto P, Molina F, Poggi S, Davenport M, Nicolaides KH. Prenatal diagnosis and outcome of echogenic fetal lung lesions. Ultrasound Obstet Gynecol 2008;32:769-83.

49- Pinto RM, Araujo Junior E, Augusto LC, Costa JI, Dias DA, Aguiar LB et al. Spontaneous regression of intralobar pulmonary sequestration during the pregnancy: report of two cases through relationships between mass and fetal biometry and review of the literature. J Matern Fetal Neonatal Med 2016;29:1720-4.

51- Andrade CF, Ferreira HP, Fischer GB. Congenital lung malformations. J Bras Pneumol 2011;37:259-71.

52- Kim HK, Choi YH, Ryu SM, Chae YS, Sohn YS, Kim HJ. Infected infradiaphragmatic retroperitoneal extralobar pulmonary sequestration: a case report. J Korean Med Sci 2005;20:1070-2.

53- Fabre D, Rohnean A, Fadel E, Dartevelle PG. Giant aneurysmal dilation of an intralobar pulmonary sequestration artery. Eur J Cardiothorac Surg 2009;36:413-4.

54- Yamasaki M, Suzuki M, Misumi H, Abe K, Ito J, Kawazoe K. Hybrid surgery for intralobar pulmonary sequestration with aortic aneurysm. Ann Thorac Surg 2014;98:e11-3.

55- Chatelain S, Comp RA, Grace RR, Sabbath AM. Cardiomyopathy Induced by Pulmonary Sequestration in a 50-Year-Old Man. Tex Heart Inst J 2015;42:63-5.

56- Li X, He W, Li J, Ouyang R, Chen P, Peng H, et al. Pulmonary sequestration associated with increased serum tumor markers and elevated standard uptake

value level in PET/CT: A case report and literature review. Medicine 2018;97:e11714.
57- Shiota Y, Kitade M, Furuya K, et al. A case of intralobar pulmonary sequestration with high serum CA19-9 levels. Acta Med Okayama 1988;42:297-300.
58- Dong J, Cai Y, Chen R, Du S, Chen Y, Shi K. A case report and a short literature review of pulmonary sequestration showing elevated serum levels of carbohydrate antigen 19-9 J Nippon Med Sch 2015;82:211-5.
59- Yoshitake S, Hayashi H, Osada H, Kawahara M. Emergency laparotomy helped the resection of an intralobar pulmonary sequestration with haemorrhagic shock. Euro J Cardio-Thorac 2013;43:190-2.
60- Witlox RS, Lopriore E, Walther FJ, Rikkers-Mutsaerts ER, Klumper FJ, Oepkes D. Single-needle laser treatment with drainage of hydrothorax in fetal bronchopulmonary sequestration with hydrops. Ultrasound in Obstetrics & Gynecology: Ultrasound Obstet Gynecol 2009;34:355-7.
61- Ruano R, de A Pimenta EJ, Marques da Silva M, Maksoud JG, Zugaib M. Percutaneous intrauterine laser ablation of the abnormal vessel in pulmonary sequestration. J Ultrasound Med 2007;26:1235-41.
62- Nicolini U, Cerri V, Groli C, Poblete A, Mauro F. A new approach to prenatal treatment of extralobar pulmonary sequestration. Prenat Diagn 2000;20:758-60.
63- Bermudez C, Perez-Wulff J, Bufalino G, Sosa C, Gomez L, Quintero RA. Percutaneous ultrasound-guided sclerotherapy for complicated fetal intralobar bronchopulmonary sequestration. Ultrasound Obstet Gynecol 2007;29(5):586-9.
64- Anandakumar C, Biswas A, Chua TM, Choolani M, Chia D, Wong YC et al. Direct intrauterine fetal therapy in a case of bronchopulmonary sequestration associated with nonimmune hydrops fetalis. Ultrasound in Obstetrics & Gynecology: Ultrasound Obstet Gynecol 1999;13(4):263-5.
65- Adzick NS, Harrison MR, Crombleholme TM, Flake AW, Howell LJ. Fetal lung lesions: management and outcome. Am J Obstet Gynecol 1998;179:884-9.
66- Grethel EJ, Wagner AJ, Clifton MS, Cortes RA, Farmer DL, Harrison MR et al. Fetal intervention for mass lesions and hydrops improves outcome: a 15-year experience. J Pediatr Surg 2007;42:117-23.
67- Zhou H, Tang S, Fu Q, Yu L, Liu L. Hybrid surgery in treatment of pulmonary sequestration with abdominal aorta feeding vessel: a case report. J Cardiothorac Surg 2018;13:44.
68- Zhang N, Zeng Q, Chen C, Yu J, Zhang X. Distribution, diagnosis, and treatment of pulmonary sequestration: Report of 208 cases. J Pediatr Surg 2019;54:1286-1292.

69- Brown SC, De Laat M, Proesmans M, De Boeck K, Van Raemdonck D, Louw J et al. Treatment strategies for pulmonary sequestration in childhood: resection, embolization, observation? Acta Cardiol 2012;67:629-34.
70- Shen JF, Zhang XX, Li SB, Guo ZH, Xu ZQ, Shi XS, et al. Complete videoassisted thoracoscopic surgery for pulmonary sequestration. J Thorac Dis 2013;5:31-35.
71- Yasser A K. Contemporary Management of Pulmonary Sequestration. Open Access J Surg 2018;9:555756.
72- Bal S, Elshershari H, Celiker R, Celiker A. Thoracic sequels after thoracotomies in children with congenital cardiac disease. Cardiol Young 2003;13:264-7.
73- Findik G, Gezer S, Sirmali M, Turut H, Aydogdu K, Tastepe I et al. Thoracotomies in children. Pediatr Surg Int 2008;24:721-5.
74- Shen JF, Zhang XX, Li SB, Guo ZH, Xu ZQ, Shi.XS, et al. Complete video-assisted thoracoscopic surgery for pulmonary sequestration. J Thorac Dis 2013;5:31-35.
75- Rothenberg SS. First decade's experience with thoracoscopic lobectomy in infants and children. J Pediatr Surg 2008;43:40:4.
76- Motono N, Iwai S, Funasaki A, Sekimura A, Usuda K, Uramoto H. Indocyanine green fluorescence-guided thoracoscopic pulmonary resection for intralobar pulmonary sequestration: a case report. J Med Case Rep 2019;13:228.
77- Albanese CT, Sydorak RM, Tsao K, Lee H. Thoracoscopic lobectomy for prenatally diagnosed lung lesions. J Pediatr Surg 2003;38:553-5.
78- Bal S, Elshershari H, Celiker R, Celiker A. Thoracic sequels after thoracotomies in children with congenital cardiac disease. Cardiol Young 2003;13:264-7.
79- Liu C, Pu Q, Ma L, Mei J, Xiao Z, Liao H, et al. Video-assisted thoracic surgery for pulmonary sequestration compared with posterolateral thoracotomy. J. Thorac Cardiovasc Surg 2013;146:557-61.
80- Choudhury SR, Chadha R, Mishra A, Kumar V, Singh V, Dubey NK. Lung resections in children for congenital and acquired lesions. Pediatr Surg Int 2007;23:851-859.
81- Guys JM, De Lagausie P. Surgical techniques for pulmonary exeresis in children. In: XXIII [eme]pediatric visceral surgery teaching seminar. La chirurgie thoracique de l'enfant. Nancy;2004. p.21-34.
82- Brouchet L, Marcheix B, Renaud C, Berjaud J, Dahan M. Partial pulmonary exereses. EMC, Techniques chirurgicales-thorax, 42 350,2005.
83- Inoue T, Oizumi H, Nakamura M, Sadahiro M. Port-Access Thoracoscopic

Anatomical Segmentectomy for Pediatric Intralobar Pulmonary Sequestration. Thorac Cardiovasc Surg Rep 2014;3:42-4.
84- Yucel O, Gurkok S, Gozubuyuk A, Caylak H, Sapmaz E, Kavakli K. Diagnosis and surgical treatment of pulmonary sequestration. Thorax Cardiovasc Surg 2008;2013:154-7.
85- Zener R, Bottoni D, Zaleski A, Fortin D, Malthaner RA, Inculet RI, et al. Transarterial embolization of intralobar pulmonary sequestration in a young adult with hemoptysis. J Thorac Dis 2017;9:E188-E193.
86- Yoon HM, Kim EA, Chung SH, Kim SO, Jung AY, Cho YA et al. Extralobar pulmonary sequestration in neonates: The natural course and predictive factors associated with spontaneous regression. Eur Radiol 2017;27:2489-96.
87- Healy J, Healey A, Kitley C. Embolization of symptomatic intralobar pulmonary sequestration - A minimally invasive treatment option. Radiol Case Rep 2019;14:759-62.
88- Endovascular treatment of pulmonary sequestration with thoracic endograft: Two case reports: Erratum. Medicine (Baltimore) 2019;98:e17603.
89- Park ST, Yoon CH, Sung KB, Yoon HK, Goo DE, Kim KS et al. Pulmonary sequestration in a newborn infant: treatment with arterial embolization. J.Vasc Interv Radiol 1998;9:648-50.
90- Adelman RD, Morrell RE. Coarctation of the abdominal aorta and renal artery stenosis related to an umbilical artery catheter placement in a neonate.Pediatrics. 2000;106:E36.
91- Stanton M, Davenport M. Management of congenital lung lesions. Early Hum Dev 2006;82:289-95.
92- Gottschalk I. Strizek B. Mallmann M.R. Muller A. Geipel A. Gembruch U et al. Outcome of Bronchopulmonary Sequestration with Massive Pleural Effusion after Intrafetal Vascular Laser Ablation. Fetal Diagn Ther 2018;44:149-55.
93- Goldstein RB. A practical approach to fetal chest masses. Ultrasound Q. 2006;22:177-94.
94- Wani SA, Mufti GN, Bhat NA, Baba AA. Pulmonary Sequestration: Early Diagnosis and Management. Case Rep Pediatr 2015; 454860.
95- Zoeller C, Ure BM, Dingemann J. Perioperative Complications of Video-Assisted Thoracoscopic Pulmonary Procedures in Neonates and Infants. Eur J Pediatr Surg 2018;28:163-170.
96- Cheng K, Yuan M, Xu C, Yang G, Liu M. A chest tube may not be necessary in children thoracoscopic lobectomy. Medicine (Baltimore) 2019;98:e15857.

97- Pefoubou Y, Galloy MA, Mainard L, Pecastaings M, Antunes L, Demiscault G. Lung sequestrations: contribution of new imaging techniques in the fetus and neonate. Feuill Radiol 2005; 45:97-106.

98- Michaux H, Noel JB, Besnard M, Prevot M, Sauvage PJ. Extra-lobar sequestration associated with a bronchogenic cyst. A case report. J Radiol 2010;91:1164-7.

99- Ko SF, Ng SH, Lee TY. Noninvasive imaging of broncho-pulmonary sequestration. Am J Roentgenol 2000;175:1005-12.

100- C Hafsa, M Belguith, M Golli, H Rachdi, S Kriaa, A Elamri et al. Imagerie du cyst hydatique du poumon chez l'enfant. Editions Francises de Radiologie 2005;86:405-10.

101- Nagasaka S, Kina S, Arimoto Y, Yokote F, Uchida T, Matsubara H. Rare localized extralobar sequestration with congenital cystic adenomatoid malformation: a case report. Surg Case Rep 2017 ;3:47.

102- de Lagausie P, Bonnard A, Berrebi D, Petit P, Dorgeret S, Guys JM. Video-assisted thoracoscopic surgery for pulmonary sequestration in children. Ann. Thorac. Surg 2005 Oct; 80 (4): 1266-9.

103- Alsumrain M, Ryu JH. Pulmonary sequestration in adults: a retrospective review of resected and unresected cases. BMC Pulm Med 2018;18:97.

104- Berna P, Cazes A, Bagan P, Riquet M. Intralobar sequestration in adult patients. Interac Cardiovasc Thorac Surg 2011;12(6):970-2.

105- Albanese CT, Rothenberg SS. Experience with 144 consecutive pediatric thoracoscopic lobectomies. J Laparoendosc Adv Surg Tech A 2007;17:339-41.

106- Kumar B, Agrawal LD, Sharma SB. Congenital bronchopulmonary malformations: a single-center experience and a review of literature. Ann Thorac Med. 2008;3:135-9.

107- Shanmugam G, MacArthur K, Pollock JC. Congenital lung malformations--antenatal and postnatal evaluation and management. Eur J Cardiothorac Surg 2005 ;27:45-52.

108- Tocchioni F, Lombardi E, Ghionzoli M, Ciardini E, Noccioli B, Messineo A. Long-term lung function in children following lobectomy for congenital lung malformation. J Pediatr Surg 2017;52:1891-7.

109- Lau CT, Wong KK. Pediatric minimal invasive surgery- thoracoscopic lobectomy. Ann Laparosc Endosc Surg 2018;3:94.

List of abbreviations

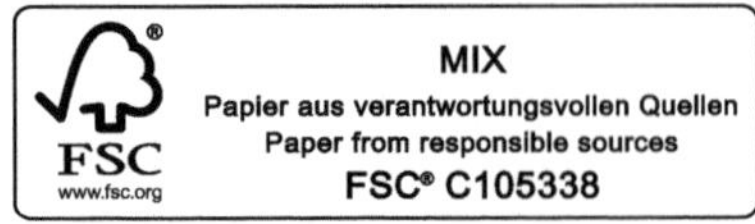

Printed by Books on Demand GmbH, Norderstedt / Germany